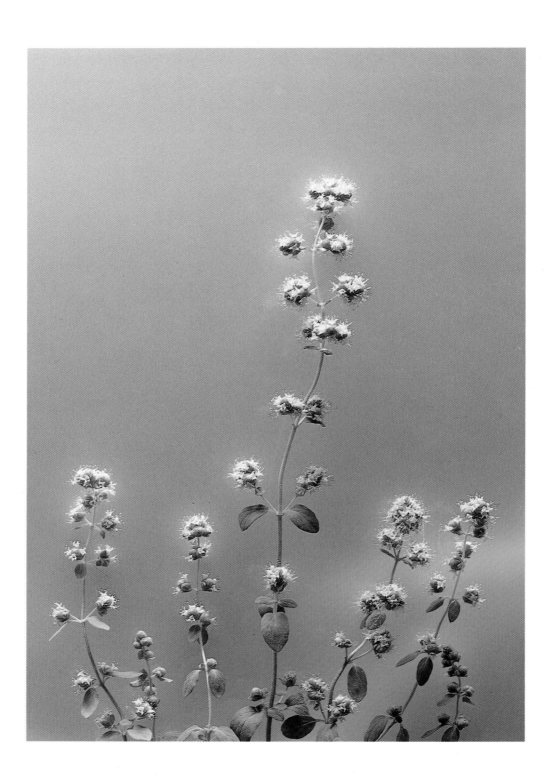

AROMATHERAPY
— *for* —
COMMON AILMENTS

Shirley Price

A GAIA ORIGINAL

615
PRIC
C. I

A Fireside Book
Published by Simon & Schuster Inc.

A GAIA ORIGINAL

Conceived by   Joss Pearson

Editorial   Gian Douglas Home
Design   Helen Spencer

Photography   Philip Dowell
                    Fausto Dorelli

Illustration   Ann Chasseaud
Reference
    photography   Jeremy Gunn-Taylor

Direction   Joss Pearson
                    Bridget Morley

FIRESIDE
Simon and Schuster Building
Rockefeller Center
1230 Avenue of the Americas
New York, New York 10020

Typeset by Tradespools Ltd., Somerset, UK
Reproduction by Fotographics Ltd., Hong Kong
Printed and bound by Kyodo Ptg Singapore Pte Ltd

Library of Congress Cataloging-in-Publication Data
Price, Shirley.
    Aromatherapy for common ailments/Shirley Price.
        p.   cm.
    "A Fireside book."
    "A Gaia original" – T.p. verso.
    Includes bibliographical reference and index.
    ISBN 0-671-73134-3
    1. Aromatherapy.   I. Title.
RM666.A68P75   1991
615'.321 – dc20

ISBN: 0-7432-5412-0

10 9 8 7 6 5 4 3 2 1

How to Use This Book

Whether you intend to use essential oils on a regular basis
for pleasure and to prevent ill health or for the relief of a
particular health problem, you should first familiarize
yourself with chapter 2 *How to Use Home Treatments*, which
gives clear guidelines on how to dilute and blend the oils
for home use and the different methods of application.
Chapter 3 *Everyday Aromatherapy* will provide you with
innovative ideas on preventative aromatherapy – how to use
essential oils about the home to improve hygiene, prevent
ill health, and maintain physical vitality and emotional
equilibrium. For advice on self-help aromatherapy, turn to
chapter 4 *The Ailments* which covers over 40 common
health problems (grouped under mind and body systems
for ease of reference) and gives dosage and treatment
instructions for the therapeutic use of 30 different essential
oils. (For detailed instructions on preparing and applying
essential oils, refer back to chapter 2.) Chapter 4 also
contains special features on 12 of the most versatile
essential oils for home use. In chapter 1 *The Nature of
Aromatherapy*, you will find details on the production,
composition, and therapeutic value of essential oils,
together with a chart (pages 14 to 15) which allows you to
see at a glance which oils are recommended for a particular
ailment. Before buying or using essential oils, read the
cautions on the use of certain oils given opposite.

Notes to the reader:

The predicted benefits of aromatherapy are not so much
based on conventional scientific study as on the
observations of practitioners over many years of practice.
Thus, where the text in the book makes claims, for
example, that a certain essential oil has anti-viral
properties, it normally means that this improvement has
been observed in practice. While critics might call it
coincidence, aromatherapists feel that the results occur
frequently and consistently enough to represent true
therapeutic effects. Although some essential oils have
undergone laboratory testing, many more have yet to be
scientifically examined.

The techniques, ideas, and suggestions in this book are not
intended as a substitute for proper medical advice. Any
application of the techniques, ideas, and suggestions in this
book is at the reader's sole discretion and risk.

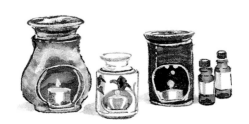

Cautions on the use of essential oils

The oils recommended in this book have been carefully selected for their gentle healing properties. Their chemical composition is such that they present no risk of toxicity, provided you adhere to all dosage instructions and follow any cautionary advice closely. Pay particular heed to children's dosages (page 88).

Some essential oils have stronger powers and can be toxic if used in their undiluted state over a prolonged period; you should use these oils only under the guidance of a professional aromatherapist or medical herbalist (see list B). A few essential oils are extremely powerful and are not meant for use in aromatherapy. Although these oils are supplied mainly to pharmacists, herbalists, perfumers, and food manufacturers, a few are available to the general public (see list A). Do not attempt to use these yourself. When choosing essential oils, bear in mind the following points:

○In some instances, a whole plant may be safely used by a herbalist, but its essential oil, containing a higher concentration of natural chemicals, may not be recommended for use in aromatherapy.

○Most health-food stores supply quality essential oils, but be sure to buy only those that are clearly labelled "pure essential oil".

○Where the oil of a specific variety is recommended, only purchase it from a vendor who knows the full latin name of the plant from which the oil is distilled. See page 14 for latin names of all oils recommended in this book.

○If you suffer from high blood pressure, epilepsy, or a progressive neural disorder, the actions of some essential oils may adversely affect your condition. Before use, consult a professional aromatherapist or medical herbalist. For oils that are best avoided in early pregnancy, see List C.

List A

The following oils are best not used in aromatherapy because of their potentially toxic nature and strong emmenagogic (ability to induce menstruation) action: American Pennyroyal *Hederoma pulegoides*, Mugwort *Artemisia vulgaris*, Pennyroyal *Mentha pulegium*, Rue *Ruta graveolens*

List B

When employed incorrectly, the following oils can have adverse effects and so should only be used under the guidance of a professional aromatherapist: Aniseed *Pimpinella anisum*, Bay *Pimenta racemosa*, Camphor *Cinnamomum camphora*, Carrot seed *Daucus carota*, Cinnamon *Cinnamomum zeylanicum*, Clove *Eugenia caryophyllata*, Hyssop *Hyssopus officinalis*, Lemongrass *Cimbopogon citratus*, Sage *Salvia officinalis*, Savory *Satureia hortensis*, Tarragon *Artemisia dracunculus*, Thyme *Thymus vulgaris*

List C

In early pregnancy, it is best to avoid emmenagogic oils that may induce menstruation, and those with diuretic properties, which can deplete fluid in the foetal sac. Consequently, you should avoid the following during the first five months of pregnancy:
Angelica *Angelica archangelica*, Clary Sage *Salvia sclarea*, Juniper Berry *Juniperus communis*, Lovage *Levisticum officinale*, Rosemary *Rosmarinus officinalis*, Spanish Marjoram *Thymus mastichina*, Sweet Marjoram *Origanum majorana*, Sweet Fennel *Foeniculum vulgare*, True Melissa *Melissa officinalis*

Note: Essential oils of Lavender *Lavandula officinalis* and Roman Chamomile *Anthemis nobilis* are very gentle emmenagogues; Lavender is also a mild diuretic. You can, however, use both of them in early pregnancy, unless you have a history of miscarriage, when it is safer to exclude them.

List D

The following oils can cause skin photosensitization to ultraviolet rays from the sun and other sources. Avoid exposure to ultraviolet rays for a minimum of four hours following treatment.
Angelica *Angelica archangelica*, Bergamot *Citrus bergamia*, Bitter Orange *Citrus aurantium amara*, Lemon *Citrus limon*, Lime *Citrus aurantifolia*, Mandarin *Citrus reticulata*, Sweet Orange *Citrus sinensis*

Contents

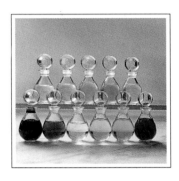

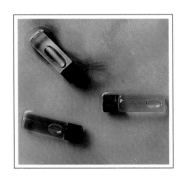

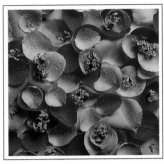

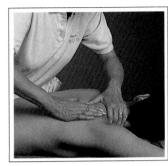

Introduction

Aromatherapy makes us aware of the need to develop our sense of smell if we are to benefit fully from the riches of the natural world. The aromas emanating from plants are often due to the presence of powerful healing substances, essential oils, that can help us in times of trouble when our physical or mental balance is disturbed. These potent, volatile essences, hidden in tiny glands within the plant, contain many beneficial properties and are used in aromatherapy to increase vitality and health.

Aromatic herbs have been used since antiquity to cleanse and heal both body and mind. Records from the East indicate that primitive stills were employed as far back as 5000 years ago, although probably more for the production of aromatic waters than essential oils. In ancient Egypt, aromatic waters and resins featured in ceremonies and rituals, while the rich perfumed themselves with scented ointments, made by infusing aromatic plants in oily or fatty substances. In the embalming process, oils of cedarwood and frankincense were used, no doubt for their preserving properties, to impregnate the bandages of mummies. How much the ancients knew of the plants' healing powers is uncertain, but ayurvedic medical texts from early Indian society include aromatic essences in many of their treatments. Subsequent civilizations, notably the Greeks and Romans, developed the use of these essences in rituals and religious ceremonies and records indicate an increasing awareness of their therapeutic properties. By AD 1000, the Arab physician Avicenna had introduced the cooling system into the distillation process, making the extraction of essential oils a more refined and efficient process.

An indication of the antiseptic properties of what we now know as essential oils came from the apparent immunity of many perfumers to the plagues and cholera that swept Europe during the Middle Ages, and by the late 17th century the oils were widely used in medicine. Toward the end of the 19th century, scientific experiments into the anti-bacterial properties of plants began to clarify the chemical composition and potential healing powers of essential oil molecules. Unfortunately, rather than leading to an increase in the use of essential oils, attempts were made to mimic their properties and, increasingly, synthetic chemical equivalents were employed instead of the plant essences themselves.

The reintroduction of the use of essential oils began in the early 1900s with the work of a French chemist, René-Maurice Gattefossé, who first gave the name "aromathérapie" to this branch of herbal medicine.

Another Frenchman, Dr Jean Valnet, became interested in the healing properties of essential oils after using them to treat soldiers' wounds in World War II. His subsequent extensive coverage of the subject gained official recognition for the therapy in France, where today many doctors prescribe oils for internal and external use. The development of holistic aromatherapy (see below) as it is now practised in the UK owes much to the French biochemist Marguerite Maury. She introduced essential oils into the beauty therapy world, where they were used in conjunction with massage for their rejuvenating effects on the skin.

Over the last few years, research has accelerated at universities and hospitals throughout the world. Results have given us a much deeper knowledge of the essential oils themselves, as well as an increased awareness of their exceptional strength.

Aromatherapy and your health

Aromatherapy is ideal for self-help since it is both effective and enjoyable to use. Bathing, receiving a massage, or inhaling with essential oils can help to boost the immune system and improve health and wellbeing generally. In addition, when used as indicated, essential oils have no adverse side effects. This last factor is significant at a time when more and more people are becoming aware of the potential disadvantages of some chemical drugs – the dangers of dependency, a weakened immune system, unwanted side effects, and the fact that the body frequently builds up a resistance to them. A visit to a holistic aromatherapist will give you the added benefit of a treatment that is tailored to meet your individual needs. The therapist studies you, the patient, as a whole, taking into consideration your emotional state and mental attitude, since these are often partially responsible for physical symptoms. Essential oils are then selected and mixed to suit you as an individual.

Increasingly, in the UK, the positive effects of aromatherapy are gaining the respect of orthodox medical practitioners. Several hospices and hospitals are now encouraging nurses to use essential oils on their patients. Some also employ fully trained aromatherapists on a part-time basis, or take on volunteers where funds are not available. These are welcome developments and, perhaps, one day hospitals will use essential oils to replace chemical disinfectants. This would, at least, encourage a more relaxed, health-producing frame of mind in both nurses and patients.

In writing this book, I hope that I have introduced you to a simple, pleasurable way to keep healthy and to relieve daily stress. The nature of essential oils is such that daily use of their healing and balancing powers will help you to achieve lasting emotional and physical equilibrium.

Chapter 1

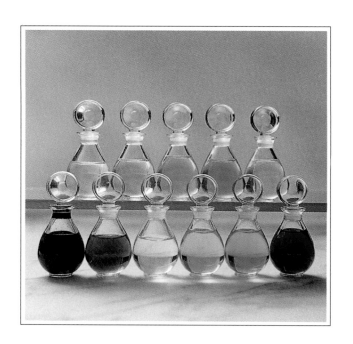

THE NATURE OF AROMATHERAPY

Like herbalism, aromatherapy draws on the healing powers of the plant world, but instead of using the whole or part of a plant, it employs only its essential oil. This potent, aromatic substance is housed in tiny glands on the outside or deep inside the roots, wood, leaves, flowers, or fruit of a plant. It is a dynamic, concentrated representation of the healing properties of the plant, and is believed by some to contain its life force. Hence care must be taken to extract the oil in its pure state.

In aromatherapy, inhalation, application, and baths are the principal methods used to encourage essential oils to enter the body. Essential oils are highly volatile, evaporating readily on exposure to air, and when inhaled, may enter the body via the olfactory system. When diluted and applied externally, essential oil molecules may permeate the skin. Bath treatments enable you both to inhale and absorb the oils. For detailed information on the main routes of entry into the body, see pages 16 to 17.

Once within your system, essential oils will work to re-establish harmony and revitalize those systems or organs where there is a malfunction or lack of balance. Their effects are many and varied (pages 16 and 93), but they are noted in particular for their antiseptic properties and their ability to restore balance to both body and mind.

A variety of factors help to determine the effectiveness of an aromatherapy treatment: the quality of the essential oils, their appropriateness for a particular individual or a specific ailment, the methods by which they are applied (pages 21 to 32), and, in the case of a professional treatment, the extent and quality of interaction between the therapist and the patient (page 33). When, for example, specialized aromatherapy massage is combined with the holistic selection of oils by a trained therapist, the effects can be truly exceptional. With self-help aromatherapy, you will be using oils recommended for a particular ailment or preventative treatment, but it should not take you long to discover which of them work best for you as an individual, particularly since simply liking the aroma of an oil may indicate that it will help you.

Producing Quality Essential Oils

To work therapeutically, essential oils need to be of the highest quality: pure, unadulterated, and, preferably, harvested from organically grown plants cultivated in optimum conditions.

When aromatic plants are produced for the perfume and food industries, the use of pesticides and fertilizers is accepted, since it gives greater and more uniform yields. For aromatherapy, natural or organic growing methods are preferred, since agrochemicals may come through in the extraction process. The altitude and soil in which the plants are grown are also important in determining the quality of the oil. Lavender raised at a high altitude on stony, dry soil yields oil of a higher therapeutic standard than that grown in rich, damp conditions on low ground. The time chosen for harvesting is significant, since it affects not only the concentration of essential oil in the plant but also its chemical composition.

The essential oil of a plant may also be affected by chemotyping, a process whereby cuttings are raised in such a way that they produce more of a desired chemical constituent. The genus of Thyme, for example, has one chemotype (for use by professional aromatherapists only) that contains a high level of carvacrol, a phenol and powerful antiseptic. By contrast, linalol, geraniol, and thujanol chemotypes of Thyme have much gentler properties. All, however, are sold under the same Latin name and, unless details are given on the label, it is best not to buy or use Thyme essential oil, since the carvacrol chemotype is the one most commonly available.

To extract essential oils in their pure state, different methods are used depending on where the essential oil is situated. With plants from the Labiatae family, such as lavender and peppermint, the essential oil glands are easily accessible, being situated on the outside of the leaves. This makes them suitable for distillation, a process in which the freshly picked or dried plant material is packed tightly into a still and steam sent through it. The heat bursts open the glands and the oil evaporates, mixing with the steam. A cooling process returns the vapours to their liquid state and the essential oil separates from the water. In the Myrtaceae family, which includes both eucalyptus and tea tree, the glands are less accessible and the plants may need bruising prior to distillation.

Citrus fruits yield their oils through hand or machine expression, which involves squeezing or scraping the rind. Where essential oil is contained in the naturally secreted resin of a plant, a solvent may be used in the extraction process. The exuded resin is dissolved in warm alcohol and filtered. The alcohol is then removed at a low temperature, leaving the resinoid: the essential oil plus a small proportion of the chemicals used.

Absolutes of rose and orange blossom are produced by a similar process; they have different chemical compositions and aromas to the pure, distilled oils of rose otto and neroli (orange blossom).

Aromatherapy users make up a negligible part of the worldwide market for essential oils. Perfume and food manufacturers, together with the pharmaceutical industry, are the main consumers. Sadly, neither of the first two is concerned primarily with purity, but rather require the oils they buy to conform to a set standard. Without adulteration, this is impossible to achieve, since essential oils are like wine – they have good and not so good years, and their aromas and flavours vary accordingly. When an oil fails to meet a customer's requirement, steps may be taken to bring it up to the required standard by adding: a poorer quality oil, a single aromatic constituent (natural or synthesized), or alcohol. As a result, sources of pure essential oils have diminished, and it is doubtful if supply will meet the increase in demand predicted for the year 2000.

Oils and their Chemistry

Essential oils have complex molecular structures and may contain up to several hundred different natural chemicals. Alcohols, esters, ketones, phenols, and aldehydes are those that feature prominently and which have been most closely studied with regard to their therapeutic potential. In general, essential oils high in alcohols and esters have gentle healing properties and are safe for home use. Ketones, phenols, and aldehydes are more powerful chemicals that are also active therapeutically. Oils that contain high concentrations of these are rarely used in aromatherapy (List B, page v), since they can have adverse effects if employed incorrectly; you should not include them in self-help treatments. A professional aromatherapist and an aromatologist, however, may prescribe them in very small doses as a means of providing speedy relief for a specific complaint.

Many of the other chemicals present in an essential oil (including the minor and, as yet, nameless ones) are thought to play a vital role in preventing side effects. Evidence for this has come from the current practice of isolating the therapeutic elements of essential oils and incorporating them in tablets and other forms of medication. The aldehyde, citral, for example, is present in lemon oil and has many beneficial effects on the body. When isolated, however, it is a very toxic substance that can cause severe skin irritation. The indication that these chemicals may contribute to the total action, or synergy, of an oil is one of the reasons why aromatherapists believe that synthetically produced equivalents cannot possibly be as effective, and that they may even be potentially hazardous.

Essential Oils and Ailments

To use the chart, either read down from the ailment until you reach a square containing a symbol, then left from there to the essential oil indicated. Or, read right from the essential oil to find out which ailments it is likely to help. For treatment instructions see pages 42 to 92. The symbols within the squares indicate which parts of the plant the oil is extracted from (see key below). The first vertical column gives the volatility (page 16) of each oil (see key below).

Essential Oil	Volatility	Mental Fatigue	Anxiety	Depression	Insomnia	Sex-drive Problems	Headaches	Throat Infections	Colds and Flu	Sinusitus	Bronchitis/Asthma	Eczema	Acne	Stretchmarks	Herpes Simplex	Athlete's Foot
Black Pepper *Piper nigrum*	●								✦							
Cajeput *Melaleuca leucadendron*	▲										✦		✦			
Caraway *Carum carvi*	△															
Cedarwood (Atlas) *Cedrus atlantica*	■							✦	✦		✦		✦			
Chamomile (Roman) *Anthemis nobilis*	●		✦	✦	✦		✦					✦	✦			
Clary Sage *Salvia sclarea*	△	✦	✦	✦		✦	✦									
Cypress *Cupressus sempervirens*	○						✦				✦	✦				
Eucalyptus *Eucalyptus globulus*	▲						✦	✦	✦	✦	✦				✦	
Frankincense *Boswellia carterii*	■													✦		
Geranium *Pelargonium graveolens*	●		✦	✦		✦			✦	✦		✦	✦		✦	
Ginger *Zingiber officinale*	■															
Juniper Berry *Juniperus communis*	●	✦	✦			✦						✦	✦			
Lavender *Lavandula officinalis*	●		✦	✦	✦		✦	✦	✦	✦	✦	✦	✦	✦	✦	✦
Lemon *Citrus limon*	▲							✦	✦				✦		✦	
Mandarin *Citrus reticulata*	▲															
Marjoram (Sweet) *Origanum majorana*	●		✦		✦	✦	✦				✦					
Melissa (True) *Melissa officinalis*	●		✦	✦		✦										
Myrrh *Commiphora myrrha*	■													✦		
Neroli *Citrus aurantium amara*	■		✦													
Orange (Bitter) *Citrus aurantium amara*	▲															
Patchouli *Pogostemon patchouli*	■															
Peppermint *Mentha piperita*	△						✦	✦	✦	✦	✦					
Petitgrain *Citrus aurantium amara*	▲												✦			
Pine *Pinus sylvestris*	●										✦					
Rosemary *Rosmarinus officinalis*	●	✦					✦		✦							
Rose Otto *Rosa centifolia, R. damascena*	■		✦	✦	✦	✦										
Sandalwood *Santalum album*	■		✦	✦	✦	✦		✦			✦	✦				
Tagetes *Tagetes glandulifera*	■															✦
Tea Tree *Melaleuca alternifolia*	▲								✦	✦		✦				✦
Ylang Ylang *Cananga odorata*	■		✦	✦	✦	✦										

KEY – ▲ = top note   △ = top to middle note   ● = middle note   ○ = middle to base note   ■ = base note

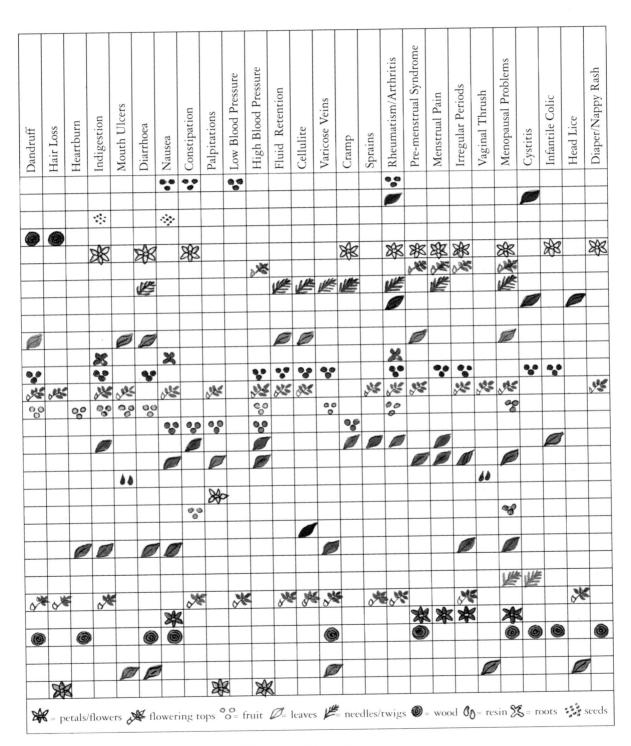

The Nature of Aromatherapy

Pathways and Effects

Holistic aromatherapists believe that essential oils enter and affect the mind and body by two principal routes – the olfactory system and the skin. Researchers have yet to provide scientific proof of this, although study on olfaction and the effects of oils on the mind is currently going on in universities in both the UK and USA. It is thought that essential oils work as triggers on the central nervous system when inhaled, and that they permeate through to the capillaries and cell tissues when applied to the skin (see opposite).

Observations of the effectiveness of essential oils are gradually being backed by studies taking place in parts of central Europe, the USA, Australia, and the UK. All essential oils appear to be antiseptic and bactericidal to some degree, and some may also be helpful in the treatment of viral infections, which are resistant to all known orthodox medicines. Many essential oils have the potential to stimulate healthy cell renewal and growth, and to regulate and restore balance to mind and body systems. Essential oils are noted too for their ability to relieve stress and stimulate sluggish circulation. These qualities, combined with their regenerative powers, give strength to claims that they can boost the immune system (page 35). Individually, they may be active on the body in a range of ways: relieving pain, reducing swelling, or cleansing impurities – to name but a few. For more detailed information, turn to the Glossary on page 93.

The beneficial effect that essential oils can have on the mind lends an added dimension to their use in healing. All essential oils help to balance the emotions to some degree, and individually they may be noted for their stimulating, uplifting, relaxing, or euphoric properties. On an intellectual level, they can revive a tired mind and stimulate the memory. Interestingly, the area of the brain associated with smell is also that in which the memory is stored and aromas have effectively been used to trigger the minds of those suffering from amnesia.

Volatility

Perfumers classify essential oils by their volatility, the speed with which they evaporate when exposed to air. Accordingly, they are given top, middle, or base "notes". This classification system is of interest to aromatherapists because of the link that appears to exist between the rate of evaporation and the effect that the oils have on the mind and body. For example, top notes, the quickest to evaporate, usually uplift the mind, whereas base notes, released much more slowly, are on the whole more calming. Middle notes, with an evaporation rate between the other two, concentrate their balancing effects on the physical systems of the body.

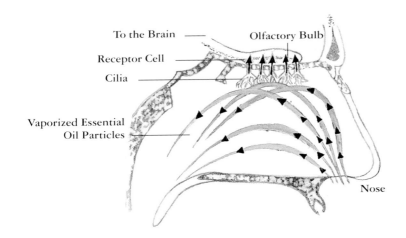

To the Brain

Receptor Cell

Cilia

Vaporized Essential
Oil Particles

Olfactory Bulb

Nose

Essential oils and olfaction

When inhaled, essential oil particles are taken directly to the roof of the nose, where the receptor cells of the olfactory system are situated. From each receptor cell protrude thin hairs (cilia) which register and transmit information about the aromas, via the olfactory bulb, to the centre of the brain. From here, electro-chemical messages are forwarded to the area of the brain associated with smell. These trigger the release of neurochemicals, which may be sedative, relaxing, stimulating, or euphoric in effect. Other messages may be relayed to parts of the body registering the oils' physical effects. Aromatic particles also travel down the nasal passages to the lungs.

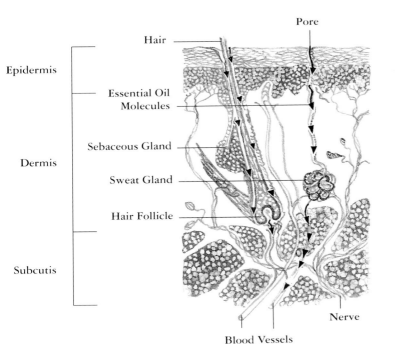

Pore

Hair

Epidermis

Essential Oil
Molecules

Sebaceous Gland

Dermis

Sweat Gland

Hair Follicle

Subcutis

Nerve

Blood Vessels

Essential oils and the skin

When dissolved in a carrier and rubbed into the skin, or when dispersed in water, tiny essential oil molecules readily permeate the skin. Via the pores and hair follicles, they can reach the fine, blood-carrying capillaries. Once in the bloodstream, they are transported round the body and filtered through to the cells and body fluids. Mucous membranes are also receptive to essential oils.

Chapter 2

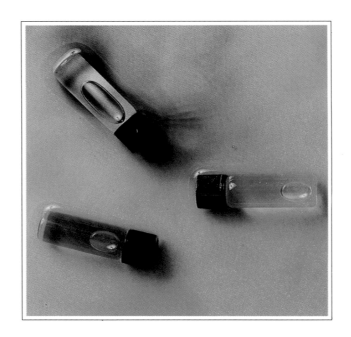

HOW TO USE HOME TREATMENTS

On the following pages, you will find clear guidelines on how best to dilute and blend your own oils, descriptions of the self-help treatments employed in aromatherapy, including illustrated massage sequences for you to share with a partner or use on yourself, and, finally, advice on when to consult a professional aromatherapist. Whether you are using aromatherapy on a regular, everyday basis (pages 34 to 41) or to treat a specific ailment (pages 42 to 92), you should read the points below carefully and also those listed at the beginning of chapter 4.

Points to Observe

○ Use only the oils recommended in this book and keep to the dosage and treatment guidelines given. For information on potentially hazardous essential oils, see page v.

○ **Never take essential oils internally on your own initiative.** Certain essential oils may be given for ingestion by a professional aromatologist, a herbalist, or a doctor.

○ **Keep essential oils away from the eyes and out of the reach of any children.** If you do get neat or diluted essential oil in your eye, rinse it out immediately with lots of water. Put some drops of sweet almond oil in the eye to dilute any remaining essential oil and to soothe irritation. (For specific advice on treating children, see page 88.)

○ Do not apply undiluted essential oils to the skin, unless specific instructions are given to do so.

○ Citrus oils are photosensitive to ultraviolet rays and may cause a skin reaction. Keep out of the sun (or other sources of ultraviolet light) for a minimum of four hours after treatment with a citrus oil.

○ If you are prone to allergic reactions, carry out the following allergy test before using an oil for the first time. Place one drop of carrier oil or lotion on your breastbone or behind your ear and leave for 12 hours. If there is no adverse reaction, dilute one drop of the essential oil in half a teaspoon of the same carrier oil or lotion, and rub the mix on your breastbone or behind your ear. Allow 12 hours for any reaction to show.

Diluting

Neat essential oils are powerful, concentrated substances. Prior to use on the skin, they are normally diluted in a carrier oil or lotion to facilitate application and to ensure against a skin reaction.

Suitable carriers

Your skin will benefit if you use cold-pressed vegetable oils as carriers, since these have healing properties and are easily absorbed. Grapeseed, sunflower, and sweet almond oils are light and easy to use. Wheatgerm, olive, and avocado oils are thicker, good for dry skin, and usually mixed with a lighter carrier oil. Macerated calendula oil, obtained by infusing the flowerheads in a carrier base, is invaluable for skin problems. Jojoba, a liquid wax, is good for all skin types.

Carrier lotion is made from emulsified oil and water. It is an ideal carrier for use in self-application since it is nongreasy. For suppliers of quality carrier lotions and oils, see *Useful Addresses* page 93.

Basic steps

Elsewhere in this book, you will find specific diluting instructions given for individual remedies, but when experimenting with your own blends, keep to the following formulae.

Essential oils		Carrier oil or lotion
20 drops	in	2fl oz (60ml/10tsp)
10 drops	in	1fl oz (30ml/5tsp)
5 drops	in	½fl oz (15ml/2½tsp)
4 drops	in	2tsp

1 When making a mixture for repeated use, choose either a 1fl oz (30ml) or 2fl oz (60ml) screw-top bottle. For ½fl oz (15ml) or less, use an eggcup.
2 Measure the carrier oil or lotion into the empty container.
3 Add the drops of essential oil. If using a bottle fasten the top securely, shake well, and label clearly.

Blending

Essential oils are synergists, complementing and enhancing each other's actions. For this reason, blends of between two and four essential oils are usually recommended for optimum therapeutic effect. To create your own blend, choose oils to suit your emotional and physical needs (see chart on pages 14 and 15), favouring those with aromas that appeal to you. Put 20 drops of each oil in a ¼oz (10 ml) brown glass, dropper bottle. Mix well and label clearly. More than four oils can be used in a blend if wished; be sure to keep a record of the number of drops of each used.

Inhalation

The inhalation of essential oils can bring speedy relief to respiratory and stress-related problems. **Caution:** Close your eyes when inhaling.

○ For immediate effect, sprinkle a total of six to eight drops of a blend of essential oils on to a tissue. Inhale deeply three times.

○ Add three to four drops of an essential oil or blend of oils to a basin of hot water. Lean over the basin, covering your head with a towel, and inhale deeply several times. **Caution:** Do not use this hot-water-based method of inhalation if you suffer from asthma, since concentrated steam can cause further breathing problems.

Baths

You can use essential oils in the bath to help a wide range of health problems. The oils do not readily dissolve in water but will disperse rapidly when swished around. Add a total of six to eight drops of one or more essential oils to a warm bath. Do not use very hot water, since this will cause the oil(s) to evaporate too quickly. If you have dry skin, dilute the essential oil(s) in two teaspoons of carrier oil before adding to the water. For maximum benefit, stay in the water for 10 to 20 minutes.

Mouthwashes and Gargles

Mouthwashes and gargles help to relieve inflamed mucous surfaces in the mouth. Add three drops of essential oil to a glass of water and stir well before taking each mouthful. Rinse out your mouth, or gargle with the liquid, before spitting it out.

Application

You can use local application to treat many skin conditions, or as an alternative to massage. Dilute the essential oil(s) in a carrier and rub well into affected areas. Keep to the diluting formulae given opposite. Unless you have very dry skin, use a nongreasy lotion as a carrier.

Compresses

An essential oil compress may soothe aches, sprains, or swelling. Cut a piece of nonmedicated lint or clean cotton to the required size. Vary the number of essential oil drops and size of receptacle according to the ailment: from two drops in an eggcupful of water for a septic finger to eight drops in a medium-sized basin of water for a wrist sprain. Use hot water for muscular aches, and cold for sprains or headaches. Immerse the cloth in the water, squeeze it lightly, and place over the affected area. Cover with plastic wrap/cling film. (Keep hot compresses warm.) Leave the compress in place for at least two hours.

Massage

Massage is used in aromatherapy both to assist the passage of essential oils into the body and to accentuate their therapeutic effects. Alone, massage can relax the muscles, enabling the blood and lymph to flow more freely, and soothe the mind. When these benefits are combined with the healing powers of essential oils, the results can be outstanding. On a physiological level, an aromatherapy massage can increase energy levels reduce stress-related symptoms, relieve pain, and, as a bonus, improve the condition of your skin. It can also restore balance to the mind by bringing about the release of such negative emotions as fear, hate, anger, jealousy, sorrow, or frustration.

Preparing for a session

The room in which you give or receive a massage needs to be comfortably warm. Use a mid-thigh level table, suitably padded, or buy a massage bed if you are anticipating regular sessions. Alternatively, make use of the floor, if you do not find that sitting or kneeling hinders your movements. Prepare your mix of oils, keeping to the dilution formulae given on page 20. For ideas on massage blends for everyday use, see page 41.

Before you give a massage, it is often a good idea to spend a few quiet moments breathing deeply to release any inner tension you may be feeling. Touch with capable and caring hands is healing in itself, and if you are also calm and able to transmit love and concern, the receiver will gain additional benefit from these positive energies. In addition, the reciprocal nature of massage is such that you as the giver should experience a pleasure equal to that of the receiver.

When fully relaxed, pour a little of the prepared blend of oils into your palm and rub your hands briefly together in order to warm and evenly distribute the oil. Bear in mind that all skins differ in absorbency and make allowances for this when applying the oil. Half a teaspoonful should be adequate for an average-sized back, but for a large, hairy, or dry back, you may need as much as a teaspoonful. Concentrate on working with the whole palm of each hand, rather than the fingers, and keep your nails short, since at times you need to use the pads of your fingers and your thumbs. It is a good idea to keep your friend's body warm by covering with a towel the parts that are not being massaged.

When there is nobody available to give you a massage, you can use basic strokes on yourself to encourage relaxation or to relieve specific problems, such as shoulder tension and varicose veins. It is easy to pinpoint tension nodules on yourself and to know how much pressure to apply, although you are restricted as to how much of your body you can reach.

Basic Strokes

For an aromatherapy massage, you need only to learn three types of basic massage stroke: effleurage, kneading, and frictions. Some variations are necessary over pressure points and to assist lymph drainage, but for those instructions are given. Never use hacking, cupping, or other staccato movements. Concentrate on effleurage strokes for general relaxation. For muscular tension, an equal amount of effleurage, kneading, and frictions is indicated.

Effleurage

The long, smooth strokes of effleurage should be used at the beginning and end of every session, and between any other type of movement. The pressure applied varies according to the direction of the stroke. Deep stroking (above), involving a firm, even pressure, is always directed toward the heart to assist the blood on its return journey. Light, gliding strokes are used when working away from the heart and to spread oil evenly over the body.

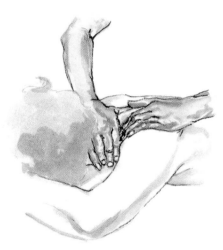

Kneading

This stroke is used to break down muscle tension and to stimulate circulation. Palms and finger lengths, or pads of fingers and thumbs, are used. Both hands work together in a rhythmic sequence, alternately picking up and gently squeezing the tense muscle, while maintaining constant contact with the skin. This results in a kneading movement, as one hand releases the muscle and the other takes over. Knuckling (p. 29) is a variation of this stroke.

Frictions

*Friction strokes are used to penetrate deep muscle tissue. The heel of the hand, or the pads of the fingers or thumbs may be used. Thumb pressure is often most effective for breaking down knotted muscle. Circular pressure may be maintained over a point, or the thumb may be guided in a wider spiral of circles. **Caution:** Never use this stroke on sciatic pain, since it can irritate the nerve.*

RECIPROCAL MASSAGE
Shoulders and Neck Massage

The following sequence is used to relieve headaches, release shoulder tension, and promote general relaxation Applying firm pressure with the thumb (b) over hard tension nodules in the shoulder and neck will help to relax knotted muscles and stimulate a general release of tension throughout the body.

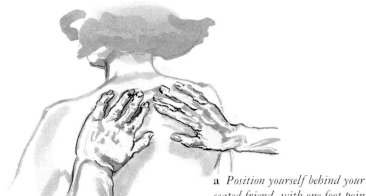

24

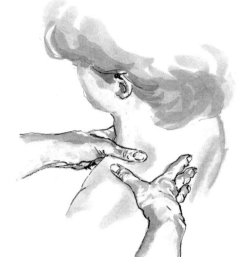

b Stand at a right angle to the side of your friend's body. Search for tension spots in the shoulder with your thumbs. Work over any that you find with alternate thumbs, using the full length of the cushioned pads. Apply sufficient pressure to reach your friend's pain threshold, but take care not to surpass it. Where you find a bad tension nodule, circle firmly with your thumb for a few seconds over the area.

a Position yourself behind your seated friend, with one foot pointing forward and the other at a right angle just behind it. Begin with effleurage, using both hands and applying firm pressure. Work from the bottom of the shoulder blades up each side of the spine to the base of the neck. Move your hands apart across the top of the shoulders and then bring them lightly down to the starting point. Repeat several times, finishing with a light return stroke.

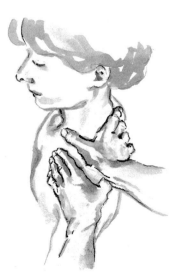

c Place your left hand in an "L" shape on your friend's shoulder. Using firm pressure, move it slowly up the whole length of the shoulder. Repeat with your other hand. Continue repeating the sequence, using alternate hands. Place one hand at the base of the back of the neck and move it up to the hairline, gently squeezing as you go. Return with a light stroke. Repeat several times. Without removing your hands, walk round to the other shoulder and repeat b and c. Move behind your friend and repeat a several times.

Back Massage

The following sequence helps to relax the whole body when carried out smoothly, without lifting the hands from the back. Applying thumb pressure to the channels on either side of the spine (**b**) on the upper half of the back will help respiratory problems. The same stroke on the lower back can alleviate constipation and menstrual pain. Steady palm pressure (**d**) assists lymphatic drainage.

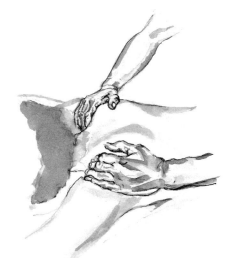

a *Place your relaxed hands, facing each other (**a**, p. 23), on either side of the base of the spine. Move them up the back, using your body weight to apply pressure. Take your hands round the shoulders (left) and return gently down the sides of the body. Repeat several times, before stopping to knead the shoulders (**b**, p. 23). Work on one shoulder, then the other. Repeat the movement.*

25

b *Position your hands at waist level, with your thumb pads in the hollows on either side of the spine, and your fingers open and relaxed. Push your thumbs firmly up the channels for 2 in (5 cm), relax them, then move them back 1 in (2.5 cm). Continue in this way up to the neck. Then gently slide both hands back to the base of the spine. Repeat. Follow with the sequence in **a**.*

c *Place your hand flat across one side of your friend's back at the base of the spine. Apply firm palm pressure and work up to the shoulders. Follow closely with your other hand. Repeat, using alternate hands. Work through the same sequence on the other side of the back, then repeat on both sides several times. Finish by working through **a**.*

d *Place your hands, facing up the back, on either side of the spine. Applying firm palm pressure, work from the base of the spine to chest level. Turn your fingers outward and move your hands apart to the sides of the body. Repeat this stroke at waist and hip levels. Repeat the first movement in **a** several times.*

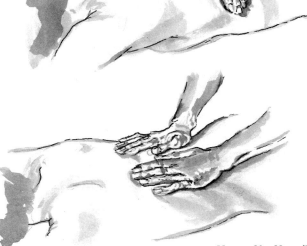

Leg, Feet, and Arm Massage

Regular leg massage can bring long-term relief to cramps. Firm upward strokes (**a**) stimulate the flow of blood and lymph and may help prevent varicose veins (**b**), while massage around the knee cap (**c**) can relieve aching. Foot massage (**d** and **e**) warms the whole body and, when combined with leg massage, is excellent for poor circulation. The arms benefit from firm upward pressure (**f** and **g**). Massage hands in a similar way to feet (**d** and **e**).

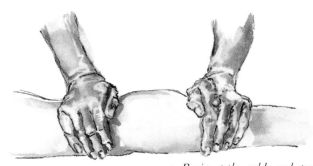

a Begin at the ankle and stroke vertically up the leg to the thigh with one hand. Follow the same path with your other hand. Continue with this sequence, using alternate hands. If your friend has varicose veins in the calves, start at the knee and work up to the thigh. Repeat several times. Then move down to the ankle and stroke up to the knee gently. Again, repeat several times.

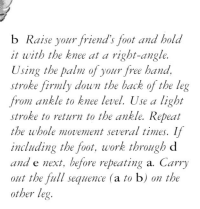

*b Raise your friend's foot and hold it with the knee at a right-angle. Using the palm of your free hand, stroke firmly down the back of the leg from ankle to knee level. Use a light stroke to return to the ankle. Repeat the whole movement several times. If including the foot, work through **d** and **e** next, before repeating **a**. Carry out the full sequence (**a** to **b**) on the other leg.*

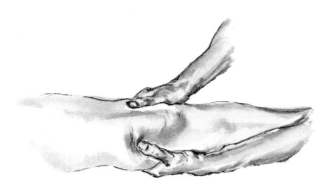

*c Help your partner to turn over and begin by stroking with alternate hands up the whole leg as in **a**. Then place your hands to either side of the knee and, using the pads of your thumbs to apply gentle pressure, circle around the knee cap. If including the foot, bring your hands down to the ankle and use the sandwich stroke (**d**) on the front of the foot. Repeat **c**. Work through the full movement on the other leg.*

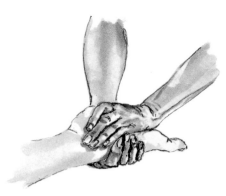

d For the following foot massage sequence, your friend should be lying face down. Take one foot between your hands, so that the palm of your upper hand is resting in the arch. Press firmly and slowly draw your hands down to the tip of the foot. Feet appreciate very firm pressure and this "sandwich" stroke gives a wonderful feeling of wholeness when used with a leg massage.

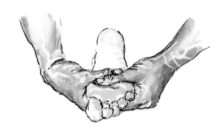

e Hold the foot with your thumbs lying side by side behind the toes. Pull both thumbs back to the sides of the foot, then push them forward. Repeating this zig-zag movement, work gradually down to the heel. Then, push firmly all the way back to the toes, keeping your thumbs side by side. Do the whole movement several times. Finish with **d**. Work through the full sequence (**d** to **e**) on the other foot.

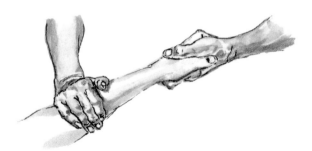

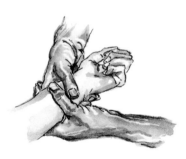

f Take hold of your friend's hand as in a firm handshake, and lift the arm up slightly, as far as the elbow. Gently place the palm of your free hand across the top of the wrist and close your fingers round the raised arm. Apply firm pressure and slide your hand up to the elbow, or as far as the shoulder. Move your palm underneath the arm and use a light stroke to return to the wrist. Repeat several times.

g Place your thumbs across the inside of your friend's wrist. Applying pressure with the pads of both your thumbs, make wide circles around the wrist area. Repeat **f** opposite. As you finish, relax your hold on the wrist and pull off firmly and slowly in a sandwich stroke, as in **d** above. Repeat the full sequence (**f** to **g**) on the other arm, finishing with the hand variation of **d**.

How to Use Home Treatments

Face and Head Massage

The following sequence encourages deep relaxation. Gentle stroking of the forehead (**b**) can help to relieve stress-related tension and headaches, while pressure applied to the sides of the nose and along the cheekbones (**c**) alleviates nasal congestion and sinus problems. Scalp massage (**d**) stimulates circulation in that area.

28

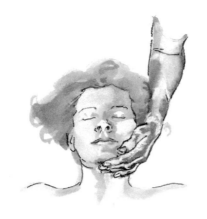

a *Use alternate hands to stroke up one side of the face, starting beneath the chin and working up toward the forehead. Work through the same movement on the other side of the face. Repeat several times. Finish by placing one palm across your friend's forehead, ready for the next stroke.*

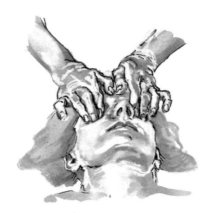

b *Begin by stroking up the forehead with alternate palms. Then, place the pads of the middle three fingers of both hands in the centre of the forehead between the eyes. Draw them gently apart across the brow and round the outside corner of the eyes. Lift off the middle two fingers and use your fourth fingers only to return under the eyes toward the nose.*

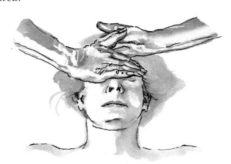

c *Position your thumbs on your friend's forehead. Using the three middle fingers of both hands, press firmly against the sides of the nose. Continue along the top of the cheekbone, until you reach the temple. Keeping your thumbs in position, return to the nose, pressing along the middle of the cheekbone.*

d *Spread out the fingers and thumbs of both hands and place them on your friend's scalp. Keep them in position and begin to move the scalp muscle over the bone by applying gentle pressure and circling slowly and firmy on the spot. Stop occasionally to move to a different area, then begin again, working gradually over the whole scalp.*

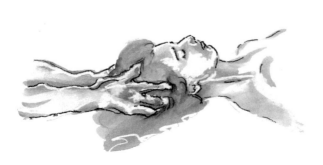

Chest and Abdomen Massage

Massage of the chest follows on naturally from the previous sequence. Knuckling (**b** and **c**) can stimulate circulation in the chest and neck areas, relax muscles in the shoulders, and may alleviate bronchial conditions. Circular pressure applied to the abdomen (**d** and **e**) can bring relief to digestive problems. The stroke used in **e** also helps menstrual pain and irregular periods.

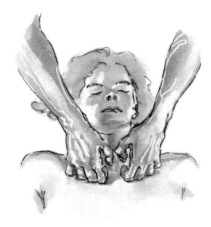

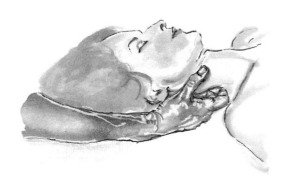

a Place both hands on your friend's chest just below the neck. Move them slowly and firmly apart across the chest until the side of each palm is lying just above the underarm crease. Continue around the arms and along the shoulders to the back of the neck. Return with a light stroke to the chest. Repeat several times. To relieve heartburn (page 64), apply circular pressure over the painful area with the heel of your palm.

b Bend your fingers inward and place the middle sections in the centre of your friend's chest. Draw your hands slowly apart toward the underarm crease. As you do so, begin knuckling by moving your fingers independently back and forth across the chest area. Without applying pressure, return your hands smoothly to the centre of the chest. Repeat.

c Bend your fingers as in b and place the middle sections under the muscle behind the shoulder. Push firmly into the muscle and pull upward while moving your fingers independently back and forth. Continue with this movement along the length of the muscle and up the neck, until you reach the base of the skull. Relax and return smoothly, without applying pressure, to the lower part of the shoulder. Repeat.

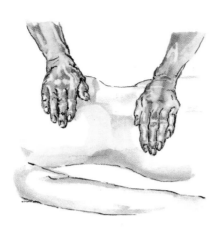

d *Place the palm of one hand on the solar plexus, the soft area that lies directly beneath the breastbone. With the palm of your other hand, move gently in a large clockwise circle round the navel. Start at the right side of the pubic bone and work up that side of the abdomen. Continue across the stomach just below the other hand, and on down the other side of the abdomen to the starting point. To relieve indigestion, make small circles with your palm wherever discomfort is felt.*

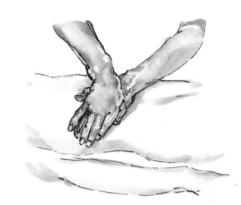

e *For a more pronounced effect, place one hand on top of the other and, keeping the fingers fully relaxed, apply firm, even pressure with your palms as you move in small clockwise circles round the abdomen. Follow the same route as in **d** above. If you concentrate on using your palms and applying firm but not heavy pressure on the upper half of each circle, your friend will benefit fully without experiencing discomfort.*

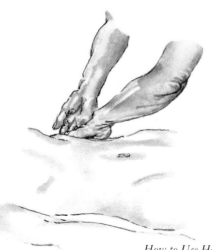

f *Start at hip level on the side of your friend's abdomen that is farthest from you, and use alternate palms to lift the body toward its centre. Continue up to chest level. Repeat several times. Bring one hand over to the near side of your friend's body and with the palm facing away from you, begin gently to lift this side of the abdomen. Follow with your other hand, and continue up to chest level, using alternate hands.*

How to Use Home Treatments

SELF-MASSAGE

When there is nobody available to give you a massage, you can use the following sequences to achieve a general release of tension. Chest massage (**e**) is good for bronchial conditions, while stroking up the leg (**g**) is an excellent treatment for varicose veins.

a *Hold your hands vertically. Place the pads of the middle three fingers of each hand on your brow between the eyes. Applying light pressure, move your hands apart across the brow to the corners of each eye. Apply gentle, circular pressure around the hollows on the outside of each eye bone (left). Use your fourth finger only, to stroke under the eyes back toward the nose. Return to the forehead and repeat the movement.*

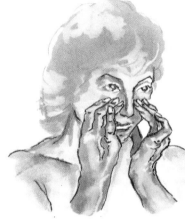

b *With your fingers pointing up and your thumbs underneath your jaw bone, press along the top of your cheekbones until you reach your temples. Return lightly to the centre. Work outward again along the middle of the cheekbone. For relief of headaches and stress-related tension, place your fingers and thumbs on your scalp and work through the movement described in **d** on page 28.*

c *Place your whole hand gently over your opposite shoulder, with your palm resting on the collar bone and your fingers resting on the shoulder muscle. Move your hand firmly along the top of the shoulder to the neck. Continue up the neck as far as you can and massage behind the ears. Return lightly to the shoulder and repeat several times.*

d *Feel with your fingers for knotty, painful areas in your shoulder muscle. Apply firm, circular pressure to any tension nodules you find, using the pads of your fingers and taking care not to exceed your own pain threshold. Keep your fingers together and remember to use the cushioned pads, not the tips. Finish off with stroke **c**. Repeat on the other shoulder.*

How to Use Home Treatments

e *Place your palm flat on your chest and, using firm pressure, make large clockwise circles. Using your fingerpads to apply pressure, continue up the neck and behind your ears. To relieve heartburn, place the pads of your middle three fingers over the painful area and, keeping them in position, move the skin over the bone. For menstrual pain and digestive problems, give yourself the abdomen massage described in* **d**, *page 30.*

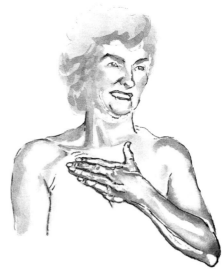

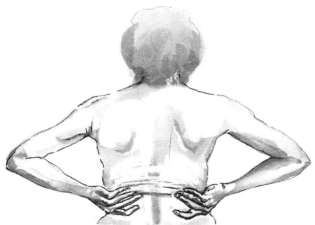

f *Sit down and place your thumbs at the front of your waist. Using your fingerpads, massage in small circles over the muscle tissue to either side of your spine. Work out toward the side of the body if necessary. If you have sciatic (nerve) pain in the lower back, try to locate the pressure points just below the hip bone, and apply pressure until the pain goes.*
Caution: *For sciatic pain, use only gentle stroking, except when working on pressure points.*

g *Place the fingers of both hands on the underside of the ankle and the thumbs on top. Stroke firmly up the leg to the knee, then use a light stroke to return to the foot. Continue with the same movement from your knee to the top of your thigh, again using a light return stroke.*
Caution: *Take care not to massage down your legs since this is not helpful to the circulation.*

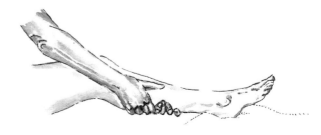

Consulting a Professional

If your symptoms do not respond to self-help treatment or if you feel that your health problem would be better treated by an expert, a visit to a professional aromatherapist should give you the improvement you desire. The therapist will carry out a holistic assessment (see below), select oils to suit you personally, and give you a treatment that may or may not include massage. If you are overwrought or fatigued as a result of stress or overwork, a full aromatherapy treatment can be immensely helpful.

Choosing a therapist

Finding a good aromatherapist is not always easy. Many people set up as professionals after only a few days' training, when in fact a minimum of six months' full-time study (18–24 part-time) is normally required before a qualifying exam may be taken. Always look out for a diploma or certificate stating that an examination has been taken; be wary of the phrase "attendance at", which usually indicates an incomplete training. If you are lucky enough to have a friend's recommendation, this is often the surest way of finding a good therapist. If not, find out whether the therapist you have chosen is a member of an aromatherapy association and selects and mixes his or her own oils. Every well-trained aromatherapist should do this and it is vital if you are to benefit fully from a treatment.

Aromatherapists do not always recommend full body massage. They may recommend part massage or may simply mix a blend for regular home use. In France, some doctors practise phytotherapy, a combination of aromatherapy and herbalism, and use essential oils differently from nonmedically qualified aromatherapists. They may prescribe intensive or internal use, as do aromatologists.

The holistic approach

On your first visit, a holistic aromatherapist will ask questions relating to your past and present state of health in order to ascertain any areas of imbalance in the mind or body which indicate a need for treatment. Your lifestyle and dietary habits may also be discussed and a range of holistic diagnostic techniques used, including testing of feet reflexes, to assess fully your condition. The therapist will then choose oils to suit your circumstances and needs. When oils are chosen in this way for you as an individual rather than just for the relief of your symptoms, the results are usually excellent and you should experience a noticeable improvement in general health and morale. Treatment may consist of up to an hour and a half of specialized aromatherapy massage, in which firm, rhythmical strokes are used. The therapist may also recommend oils for home use.

Chapter 3

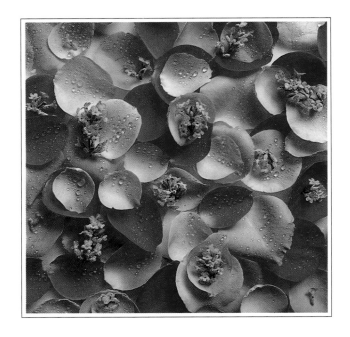

EVERYDAY AROMATHERAPY

Essential oils stimulate the senses and, when used on a regular daily basis, can significantly increase our awareness and appreciation of life. All essential oils are thought to have natural antiseptic properties, and using them in vaporizers, or as cleaning agents, will keep your home pleasantly aromatic and may also help to free it from airborne bacteria.

Incorporating essential oils into your daily routine in the form of aromatherapy skin-care products and bath and massage oils is not only pleasurable but also a means of restoring and maintaining vitality and health. Observations suggest that essential oils may be invaluable as a natural means of strengthening the body's defence mechanism, the immune system, and keeping infections at bay. The oils are believed to work in such a way that they maintain vitality and balance in all the organs and systems of the body that are actively involved in fighting invading organisms and eliminating toxins. The skin, lungs, liver, kidneys, intestines, and lymph are the principal agents of detoxification and these can benefit from the cleansing and energizing properties of many essential oils. On an emotional level, essential oils can help to bring to the surface suppressed feelings of anger, jealousy, fear, or resentment, which may eventually express themselves as physical health problems.

For essential oils to exercise their revitalizing and balancing powers to the full, however, your body and mind will need to be in a suitably receptive state. Prolonged intake of refined or processed foods, tobacco, and other pollutants, can cause toxins to accumulate in your body; a high level of stress and resultant muscular tension may impede the efficient flow of blood and lymph. Both these processes can lead to ill health. Confronted with a toxic overload and poor circulation, essential oils will concentrate their energies on relieving symptoms. To benefit you over the long term, however, they need to be combined with a relaxed and balanced lifestyle. Eating a wholesome, nutritious diet and taking positive measures to deal with stress (page 36) are therefore vital if you are to experience the full benefits and pleasures of preventative aromatherapy.

The Importance of Diet

Your daily intake of foods should consist of balanced levels of body-building proteins, energy-giving fats and carbohydrates, and the full range of vitamins and minerals. Fish is a good source of first-class protein, while seeds, peas, beans, lentils, and nuts also provide complete protein, when combined with grains. Carbohydrates are best eaten in their complex form as found in whole grains, beans, vegetables, fruit, nuts, and seeds. To obtain adequate fibre, include the pre-washed skins of fruit and vegetables. Most of the fats, minerals, and vitamins that you otherwise need are present in a varied, wholefood diet. Monounsaturated oils, found in fish, olive oil, and many nuts, are recommended, since they help to keep harmful types of cholesterol at a low level in the body. You may need to include more foods rich in vitamins C (citrus fruits, strawberries, potatoes, cabbage) and B (yeast, wheatgerm, fish, soya beans), since these are quickly used up. Green leafy vegetables, beets/beetroot, and dried fruit will provide additional iron, if required.

To complement the dietary guidelines given above, drink three or four pints of spring water daily, and eat plenty of garlic and live, natural, low-fat yoghurt. Try to avoid, or cut down on, the following items:
○ processed foods, red meat, sugar, and high levels of salt and fat
○ coffee, tea, colas, and other soft drinks that contain caffeine and/or tannin. Vary your intake of herbal teas since peppermint, maté, rose hip, yellow dock, and comfrey also contain tannin
○ alcohol, drugs, and cigarettes

Coping with Stress

Work overload, tight deadlines, difficult personal relationships, poor eating and drinking habits – any, or all, of these factors may put your system under stress. You may become anxious, depressed, or frustrated and your health and general stamina may begin to suffer as a result.

A common reaction to stressful situations is to try to escape, at least temporarily, by taking a coffee break or a quick smoke. But this only adds to the toxins in your body and does not attempt to deal with the underlying causes. A more effective tactic is to confront stress, and to tackle it positively. Reallocate your time so that more of it is devoted to enjoyable, relaxing activities and less to stress-inducing tasks. Take a short walk outside first thing in the morning, for example. Eat regularly, take time over your meals, and keep in touch with your mind and body by joining a yoga class. Last but not least, use essential oils to help you – one of their main attributes is their ability to relieve stress.

Using Oils in the Home

An important application of essential oils is around the home. As a natural alternative to chemical disinfectants, they can help to ensure household hygiene and thus go a long way to preventing ill health.

Begin by wiping down all kitchen surfaces with a cloth wrung out in a small bucket of warm water containing *4 drops each of lemon and geranium*. Scrub any wooden chopping boards once a week with the same mixture. If you wash your dishes by hand, sprinkle *2 drops each of pine and lemon or geranium and lavender* into your washing-up water. Such a small quantity of essential oil will exercise its antiseptic properties but will not leave any noticeable aroma. When washing clothes, add *3 drops each of lavender and geranium* to the final rinsing water or mix the blend with the softening agent in the rinse department of your washing machine. **Caution:** Do not use resins or absolutes (pages 12 to 13) since these can stain your clothes.

If you or a member of your family is unwell, adding essential oils to a vaporizer may help to prevent germs from spreading and stimulate recovery. For a purely preventative blend, mix together *20 drops each of tea tree, lemon, pine, and lavender* in a small brown-glass dropper bottle and add to the vaporizer (page 38) as and when required. For a more fragrant mix, use *40 drops each of geranium, lemon, and lavender*.

Catching germs from your pets is a real possibility; bear in mind that when outdoors they come into contact with litter, excreta, and other animals that may not be as clean or healthy as themselves. Most pets enjoy receiving aromatherapy treatment, but it is as well to approach with care and let your animal sniff the aroma first. When you brush your pet, dampen the bristles of the brush in a small basin of water containing *3 drops each of lemon and bitter orange and 1 drop of geranium or pine*. Squeeze out a cloth in the same mixture and use it to wipe the paws. If your pet has an infected bite, bathe it with water containing *2 drops each of tea tree and geranium*. To rid your pet of fleas, use the recipe below.

> *Anti-parasitic Blend*
> *6 drops of geranium*
> *2 drops each of lavender and tea tree*
> *1fl oz (30ml/2½tsp) of water*

Pour the water into a spray container and add the essential oils. Label the mixture clearly and shake it well before use. Ask a friend to hold your pet and shield its eyes while you gently ruffle the fur back with one hand and spray with the other.

Vaporizers and other Room Fresheners

Adding essential oils with water to a vaporizer or other type of room freshener in your living or working area will encourage aromas to linger. It will also enable you to gain maximum benefit from their antiseptic and relaxing or uplifting properties.

Vaporizers Most vaporizers are made out of clay. Some have a small loose bowl that fits on top of a type of chimney; others are of a similar structure but all in one piece. To heat the water and essential oils, insert a night light through a hole in the chimney structure; electric vaporizers are also available. To ensure that vapours continue to rise for a couple of hours, add at least four teaspoons of water to the bowl. Into this, sprinkle eight to ten drops of your chosen blend of oils. The heat will encourage evaporation and the room will gradually fill with the fragrance of the oil molecules. Replenish the bowl with essential oils and water as necessary. **Caution:** To prevent the oils burning, check that the bowl is not too near the heat source and keep an eye on the water level.

Vaporized essential oil molecules can help to eliminate airborne bacteria and make your surroundings smell wonderful, hiding unwanted odours from cigarettes, cooking, or pets. They are also invaluable as a means of balancing the emotions. A stimulating blend will clear the mind, while calming oils can relieve the tensions of a stressful day.

Choose one of the blends from below to suit your mood and circumstances. For Christmas, you can adapt the festive blend by substituting frankincense and black pepper or caraway and ginger for eucalyptus and lavender.

Restful Blend
4 drops of sandalwood
4 drops of lavender
2 drops of geranium

Festive Blend
4 drops of orange
4 drops of eucalyptus
2 drops of lavender

Light bulb ring burners These hollow, circular rings of porous clay are designed to fit over the top of a low-wattage light bulb. Position your ring on the light bulb and add eight to ten drops from your chosen blend of essential oils before you switch on the light. The heat of the bulb will vaporize the oils (do not add drops when light is on). Essential oils evaporate rapidly and may give off a burned aroma if the ring gets too hot.

Sprays For a rapid antiseptic effect, a spray is ideal since it enables you to disinfect or perfume the room with diffused essential oil molecules in seconds. Fill the spray container with water and add from eight to twelve drops of your chosen blend of essential oils. Shake before use.

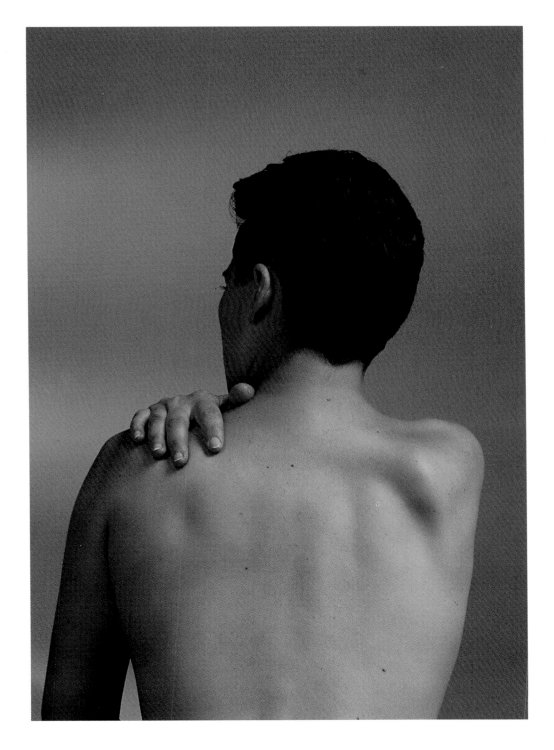

Awareness and Health

The balancing, cleansing, and regenerative qualities of essential oils are excellent for your skin. When used daily, diluted in a carrier (page 20), essential oils can improve skin texture, particularly of the face and hands – the areas most exposed to the elements. Elbows, legs, knees, and feet also take a lot of wear and tear, so don't neglect them. Make up your own range of aromatherapy moisturizing products from the recipes below for morning and evening use, and complement these with the bath and massage blends given.

Facial cleansers and toners Cleansing creams are not intended to penetrate the skin and for this reason they may contain a small proportion of mineral oil. The molecules of mineral oil are too big to be absorbed but they effectively dissolve grime and dirt. Buy a good-quality cream with no synthetic perfume or animal extracts in it from a reputable firm (see *Useful Addresses,* page 93). Those containing rosemary are good for any skin type. The toning lotion you select should not contain alcohol, since this can cause skin to become dry and patchy.

Moisturizers Moisturizers with beeswax and lanolin as their base have little beneficial effect, since they consist of molecules that are too large to penetrate the skin efficiently. By contrast, carrier lotion, made from a vegetable oil and water emulsion, is easily absorbed and makes an ideal base for an essential oil moisturizer. If you can obtain one that is free of additives, mix it with the blend below suited to your skin type.

Normal-to-oily Skin	*Dry Skin*
2 drops of juniper berry	*2 drops of lavender*
2 drops of lavender or	*2 drops each of sandalwood*
frankincense	*and patchouli*
1 drop lemon	*1 drop rose otto*
1 drop geranium	*2 tsp calendula carrier oil*
8 tsp of white carrier lotion	*6 tsp of white carrier lotion*

Make up the moisturizer for normal-to-oily skin by blending the essential oils with the carrier lotion base, and stirring well. For the dry-skin variation, add the calendula oil a little at a time to the lotion. Stir after each addition. (If your skin is very dry, you can use three rather than two teaspoons of calendula oil.) Then add the essential oils and stir well. Label the bottle containing your mixture clearly.

To make up an effective night oil for dry skin, mix *2 teaspoons each of calendula and avocado* with *5 teaspoons of sweet almond*, and add *3 drops each of sandalwood and neroli*.

Masks An essential oil face mask is easy to make up and an effective means of cleansing and revitalizing your skin. You need only apply the mask once a week to achieve a noticeable improvement in skin texture.

Normal-to-oily Skin	*Dry Skin*
2 drops of lemon	*2 drops of sandalwood*
1 drop of geranium	*1 drop of lavender*
1 drop of ylang ylang	*1 drop of Roman chamomile*
2 tsp of live, natural	*or neroli*
yoghurt	*2 tsp of honey*

Choose whichever recipe corresponds to your skin type. Blend the oils with the yoghurt or honey and spread the mixture lightly and evenly over your face and neck. After a few minutes, when the mask no longer feels cool, rinse off and apply a moisturizer.

Bath oils Make up the two blends below and keep them ready prepared. The uplifting blend will help to wake you in the morning and prepare you for the day ahead. Use the relaxing blend to relieve tension and re-store harmony at the end of a stressful day.

Uplifting Bath Oil	*Relaxing Bath Oil*
40 drops of lemon	*30 drops of petitgrain*
30 drops of black pepper	*20 drops of clary sage*
20 drops of juniper berry	*20 drops of lavender*
10 drops of peppermint	*10 drops of patchouli*

For each recipe, blend the essential oils in a brown-glass dropper bottle. Screw the bottle lid tightly shut, shake well, and label clearly. Add six to eight drops to a warm bath. For dry skin, you can dilute the essential oils in two teaspoons of carrier oil before adding to the bath.

Massage oils Use the blends below in reciprocal or self-massage (pages 24 to 32) to nourish the body and mind. The stimulating blend can help to improve poor circulation and will revive you if you are tired or run down. Keep the soothing blend for evening use, since it will relax you and prepare you for sleep.

Soothing Blend	*Stimulating Blend*
2 drops of juniper berry	*3 drops of lemon*
3 drops of lavender	*2 drops of rosemary*
2 drops of sandalwood	*2 drops of juniper berry*
1/2fl oz (15ml/2 1/2tsp) of carrier oil	*1/2fl oz (15ml/2 1/2tsp) of carrier oil*

Choose whichever blend appeals to you. Mix the essential oils with the carrier oil and store in a clearly labelled, screw-top bottle.

Chapter 4

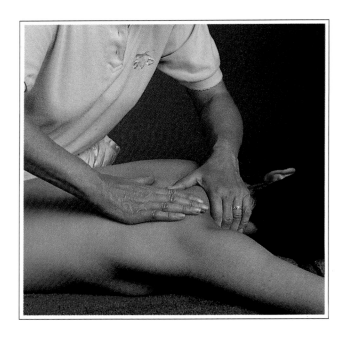

THE AILMENTS

This chapter is devoted to the therapeutic use of essential oils in the home for relief of common health problems. The oils' anti-bacterial properties can help you to fight and overcome infection and may prove invaluable in the prevention of illness; advice on their regular, daily use is given in chapter 3. In addition, many of the oils are regenerative, stimulating the healthy renewal of cells within the body, and may boost your immune system generally (page 35). This chapter tells you which oils are suitable for a particular ailment and how they are best applied, but for details on diluting and blending and the techniques involved in the different self-help treatments, you will need to refer back to chapter 2 (the relevant page number may be given to help you). All of the oils recommended have been carefully chosen and can be used successfully and without risk, provided you follow dosage and treatment instructions closely. If in any doubt, consult a professional aromatherapist.

Points to Observe
○ Never attempt self-diagnosis. If you are unsure of the cause of your symptoms, consult a medical practitioner.
○ Before using any of the treatments recommended on the following pages, read chapter 2 How to use Home Treatments (in particular the list of Points to Observe on page 19), and the cautions on the use of certain essential oils on page v.
○ If your symptoms do not respond to self-help treatment within one week, consult a professional aromatherapist or medical practitioner.
○ If you have a chronic condition and/or are taking prescribed medication, consult your doctor before using aromatherapy. Do not suddenly stop taking your medication, but if your condition improves following aromatherapy treatment, you may be able to reduce the dose you are taking under the guidance of a medical practitioner.
○ **You should never take essential oils internally on your own initiative.** However, certain essential oils may be prescribed for intensive use or ingestion by a professional aromatologist or a medical practitioner.
○ **Keep essential oils away from the eyes and out of the reach of children.** For specific advice on treating children, see page 88.

The Ailments

Emotional Problems

Positive emotions such as love and elation make us feel good, but prolonged negative feelings of fear and anxiety can depress us and endanger our health. This is because our emotions are both controlled by, and affect, the nervous system. In turn, this regulates production of the hormones needed for a balanced, healthy life. Negative reactions to everyday stresses, and the emotions we experience as a result, can block the energy flow in our bodies, cause tension in the muscles, and restrict the supply of blood and oxygen to our vital organs. Aromatherapy will help prevent and counteract these unwelcome effects by encouraging relaxation and a return to a balanced emotional state.

Mental Fatigue

This condition can result from overwork or worry over a personal problem that requires a lot of thinking through. Poor working conditions, in particular a lack of fresh air, or a shortage of vitamin B may also be instrumental in producing mental lethargy. Stress (page 36) is ofren a contributory factor, and a treatment combining relaxing and uplifting oils is often the most effective. **Caution:** If your symptoms persist, seek professional advice.

Useful Oils

Rosemary, an oil that stimulates both body and mind, is invaluable if you are mentally fatigued by overwork but need to maintain a clear head in order to complete some pressing task. Where stress is partially to blame, clary sage and juniper berry will help both to relieve tension and lift your spirits.

Treatment

Lifestyle Regular outdoor exercise is one way of keeping your mind bright and active.

Diet Eat a healthy, balanced diet (page 36) to ensure a good vitamin balance. Avoid drinking teas that contain tannin (page 36) since these hinder absorption of iron, a shortage of which can cause fatigue.

Inhalation To clear and revive a tired mind, sprinkle *a few drops of rosemary* onto a tissue. Inhale deeply. Then place the tissue inside your shirt where your body warmth will help to release the aromas.

Bath and Massage Add *3 drops each of clary sage and juniper berry* to your bath before retiring or, if you bathe in the morning, ask your partner to give you a back massage (page 25) at night, using the same blend diluted in *$\frac{1}{2}$fl oz (15ml/2$\frac{1}{2}$tsp) of carrier oil*. If alone, give yourself a shoulder massage (page 31), both night and morning. You can also put these oils in a vaporizer (page 38) during the day.

Stress-related Anxiety

For many of us, stress (page 36) and the anxiety it causes are an unavoidable part of our daily lives. A low level of stress is indeed often necessary to motivate us, but it is important to keep its impact within a level you can tolerate. If allowed to dominate, stress can cause intense anxiety and a general deterioration in health. It can also increase the risk of more serious ailments developing, such as stomach ulcers and heart disease.

Useful Oils

Many essential oils help to reduce stress by promoting relaxation, in particular the more expensive, highly aromatic ones, such as rose otto, neroli, and true melissa. Fortunately, other less expensive oils can be as effective. clary sage, geranium, Roman chamomile, juniper berry, lavender, sandalwood, sweet marjoram, and ylang ylang are all useful.

Treatment

If your emotional and physical health is already beginning to deteriorate as a result of stress, you may find it most helpful to visit a professional aromatherapist for a full treatment.

Lifestyle Take plenty of walks outdoors in the fresh air, and set aside time for relaxation and gentle exercise forms, such as yoga.

Diet Eat a healthy, balanced diet (page 36) and cut down on stimulants such as tea, coffee, and caffeinated soft drinks.

Inhalation For relief from sudden stress, sprinkle *4 drops of lavender* on to a tissue and inhale deeply.

Bath Add the *Relaxing Blend* given below to a warm bath to relieve tension.

Massage Mix the *Relaxing Blend* from the recipe with *½fl oz (15ml/2½tsp) of carrier oil*. Use the mixture in a shoulder massage (page 31) to help yourself relax or ask a friend to give you a full body massage (pages 24 to 30). Another excellent remedy for stress is simply to get someone who cares for you to hold you close. You can also use the blend below in a vaporizer (page 38) to help release tension and encourage sound sleep at the end of a stressful day.

Relaxing Blend
  2 drops of geranium
  2 drops of lavender
  2 drops of sandalwood
  1 drop of ylang ylang

Use the oils in a bath or massage, as indicated.

Depression

All of us at sometime or another suffer the misery of not wanting to get on with our lives. However, severe bouts of depression, which may be accompanied by apathy, irregular sleep patterns, loss of appetite, and generalized fatigue, can have serious effects on your health if allowed to persist. Aromatherapy treatment can be highly therapeutic but if symptoms do not improve, consult your doctor, who may recommend professional counselling.

Useful Oils

Almost all of the relaxing oils recommended opposite for stress are also good for relieving depression since they are both normalizing and uplifting. They include clary sage, Roman chamomile, geranium, lavender, rose otto, sandalwood, and ylang ylang.

Treatment

As with stress-related anxiety, a full treatment may be helpful.

Lifestyle Try to avoid spending long periods of time alone. Instead, seek out someone with whom you can talk through your feelings and any difficulties you may be experiencing.

Diet If you have the urge to eat continually, nibble healthy food, such as raw carrots and celery, rather than sweets.

Bath For a relaxing, uplifting bath, add *3 drops of clary sage, 2 drops of geranium, and 1 drop of ylang ylang* to the water.

Massage Ask one of your friends to give you a back massage (page 25) and reciprocate if you feel able to, using *2 drops each of lavender and geranium and 1 drop of Roman chamomile* mixed with *½fl oz(15 ml/2½tsp) of carrier oil*.

Inhalation Mix together *20 drops of clary sage and 10 drops of rose otto* and store the mixture in a brown glass bottle. Every morning and night, sprinkle a few drops on to a tissue and inhale. You can also use the same blend in a vaporizer (page 38), adding *2 drops of sandalwood* for a lasting effect.

Essential Oil of Clary Sage

Part of plant used: *Flowering tops*
Method of extraction: *Steam distillation*
Volatility: *Top note (page 16)*
Principal constituents: *Linalol, linalyl acetate, sclareol*

Properties, effects, and methods of use

Clary sage is both a powerful relaxant, and an energizing and invigorating essential oil. It has a pervading, sweet, sensuous aroma that can be quite heady (see caution below).

Emotional Uplifting and relaxing; helpful in relieving depression, anxiety, tension, mental fatigue, and general debility; may promote dream-filled sleep if alcohol is in the system; good for calming cross or irritable children. Used in inhalations, vaporizers, baths, application, or massage.

Respiratory Calming and anti-inflammatory; relieves sore throats and hoarseness. Used in inhalations, vaporizers, or applicaiton.

Skin Soothing and anti-inflammatory; useful for all types of skin inflammation, including boils; anti-fungal on skin; helps to preserve moisture in dry, mature skin. Used in compresses or application.

Circulatory Calming; may help reduce high blood pressure. Used in inhalations, vaporizers, compresses, baths, or massage.

Gynaecological Antispasmodic, anti-inflammatory, and a gentle menstrual stimulant; relieves pre-menstrual syndrome and menstrual pain, helps to establish menstrual regularity; soothes swollen breasts; helps to prevent hot flashes/flushes. Used in compresses, baths, or massage.

Caution: Since inhalation of the oil may cause sleepiness, keep to recommended dosages and use for short periods only, preferably at the end of the day when no further physical or mental exertion is required. Do not combine with alcohol, or inhale before driving. Avoid use during first five months of pregnancy (page v).

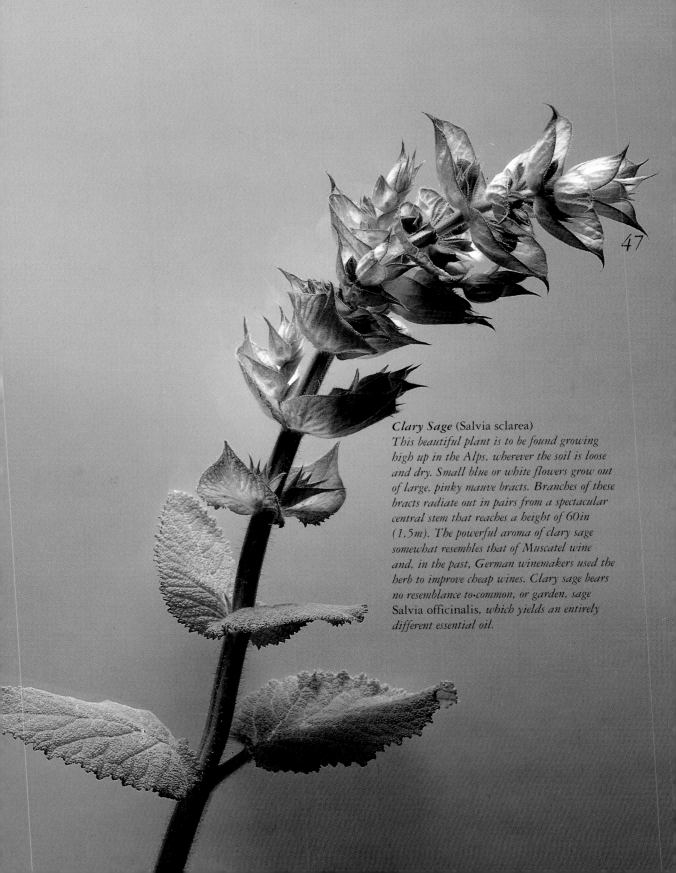

Clary Sage (Salvia sclarea)
*This beautiful plant is to be found growing
high up in the Alps, wherever the soil is loose
and dry. Small blue or white flowers grow out
of large, pinky mauve bracts. Branches of these
bracts radiate out in pairs from a spectacular
central stem that reaches a height of 60in
(1.5m). The powerful aroma of clary sage
somewhat resembles that of Muscatel wine
and, in the past, German winemakers used the
herb to improve cheap wines. Clary sage bears
no resemblance to·common, or garden, sage
Salvia officinalis, which yields an entirely
different essential oil.*

Insomnia

Insomnia may result from stress-related anxiety and tension. Other factors, such as overstimulation, or eating the wrong foods and not allowing suffcient time for digestion before going to bed, may also prevent you sleeping, with consequent worry causing recurrent sleepless nights.

Useful Oils

Oils with sedative and calming properties, such as cypress, lavender, Roman chamomile, and true melissa are the most helpful for this condition. For digestive-related insomnia, you will also need to include sweet marjoram. The addition of juniper berry, rose otto, and/or ylang ylang serves to encourage deeper sleep, as does sandalwood, another excellent remedy.

Treatment

Lifestyle Take regular outdoor exercise.
Diet Avoid stimulating drinks such as tea, coffee, and caffeinated soft drinks. Certain wines may also hinder sleep.
Inhalation Put *3 drops of lavender and 2 drops of Roman chamomile* on a tissue and inhale deeply three times (page 21). You can also sprinkle *a few drops each of lavender, Roman chamomile, and ylang ylang* on your sheets. Inhale deeply three or four times before you settle down for the night.
Bath Add the *Sleep-inducing Blend* below to an evening bath to relax you.
Massage Dilute the *Sleep-inducing Blend* below in *½fl oz (15ml/2½tsp) of carrier lotion or oil.* Use the mixture every night before you retire to massage your face and shoulders (page 31), or ask a friend to give you a regular full body massage (pages 24 to 30).

Sleep-inducing Blend
  3 drops of lavender
  3 drops of ylang ylang
  2 drops of Roman chamomile

Use the oils in a bath or massage, as indicated.

Sex-drive Problems

More often than not lack of sexual energy or desire stems from an emotional rather than a physical cause. Inbuilt fears from the past or anxiety about the present may prevent the release of, or subdue, sexual energy. Stress (page 36), and the tension and irritability that it causes, may also contribute by causing friction to develop in your relationship with your partner.

Useful Oils

The sweet, all-pervading scent of ylang ylang and the heady aroma of clary sage will help to encourage relaxation and feelings of sensuality. Rose otto, although more expensive, is another exquisitely scented oil that is closely associated with sexuality. Sandalwood and geranium are useful if you are also depressed. When selecting oils, bear in mind that an aroma which appeals to you may not necessarily be acceptable to your partner, so choose carefully, and before you blend your oils, decide what kind of effect you are after. A mixture of sandalwood and ylang ylang will give you an exotic perfume, while rose otto and geranium combined have a flowery scent. In contrast, geranium and clary sage together give off a pleasantly sharp, fresh aroma.

Treatment

Lifestyle Above all, try not to worry about your lack of sexual energy since this will only aggravate the problem. Instead, encourage yourself to relax and feel at ease with your body by indulging in gentle forms of exercise, such as swimming, outside walking, and yoga.
Inhalation To restore calm and harmony at the end of a stressful day, place one of the blends suggested above in a vaporizer (page 38) in the living room. Before going to bed, add a blend of your favourite oils to a vaporizer in the sleeping area, or sprinkle a few drops on your sheets.

Massage If your lack of sexual energy is related to stress or anxiety of some kind, gentle reciprocal massage can be a wonderful way to release tension and strengthen the bond between you and your partner. If your partner needs the treatment more than yourself, give him or her the massage first. Dilute the *Relaxing and Energizing Blend* below in *½fl oz (15ml/2½tsp) of carrier oil* and use to massage the back and abdomen (pages 25 and 30).

Bath To both relieve tension and boost your energy level, add the *Relaxing and Energizing Blend* below to an evening bath.

Relaxing and Energizing Blend
  2 drops of clary sage
  2 drops of ylang ylang
  3 drops of geranium

Use the oils in a bath or massage, as indicated.

Headaches

Tension headaches resulting from stress or overwork are common and respond well to aromatherapy rreatment. Symptoms usually include muscular tension, particularly of the scalp, shoulders, and neck. Headaches may also stem from factors such as sinus congestion, menstruation, a deficient diet, food allergy, and certain disorders of the eyes, ears, and teeth. The discomfort experienced may also give rise to tension and can similarly be eased through use of aromatherapy.

A migraine is a type of headache, typically felt on one side of the head only, that can last for two to three days. Eyesight can be affected and you may experience some nausea. Stress (page 36) or an irritant substance in your diet or environment may trigger an attack. While you may be sensitive to touch in the form of massage, inhalation can bring welcome relief.

Caution: Headaches can have more serious causes. Consult your doctor if the pain is sudden or severe, or if it recurs frequently.

Useful Oils
Lavender and sweet marjoram will both help to relieve pain, while Roman chamomile is generally soothing. For sinus congestion, add eucalyptus and/or peppermint for their decongestant properties. Sweet marjoram is particularly useful for headaches associated with menstruation, while true melissa or rosemary can help to relieve a migraine.

Treatment
Diet It is wise to seek the advice of a professional nutritionist if you think that your headache or migraine may be related to food allergy, but you can begin by excluding foods such as coffee, chocolate, cheese, and red wine, which are commonly linked with migraine attacks.

Inhalation This method can bring relief to headaches and migraines if used as soon as symptoms begin. Sprinkle *2 drops each of sweet marjoram, lavender, and peppermint* on to a tissue; for a migraine, add *1 drop of true melissa*. Inhale deeply three times.

Application To relieve a tension headache, moisten your forefinger with *2 drops of lavender* and rub gently over your temples, behind your ears, and across the back of your neck. Apply twice more, if necessary. **Caution:** Keep your fingers away from your eyes. To reduce the intensity of a headache, add *a total of 12 drops of your chosen blend to 1fl oz (30ml/ 5tsp)* of carrier oil, and apply the mix to your face and neck.

Massage Dilute *3 drops each of lavender and eucalyptus* in *½fl oz (15ml/2½tsp) of carrier oil* and use the mix to massage your forehead and behind your ears, pausing to apply gentle pressure around the hollows on the outer corners of the eye bone (illus **a**, page 31). Work along your shoulders and neck (page 31) or ask a friend to massage these areas (page 24).

Bath Add *3 drops each of sweet marjoram, Roman chamomile, and lavender* to a bath to help relieve tension headaches.

Essential Oil of Eucalyptus

Part of plant used: *Leaves*
Method of extraction: *Steam distillation*
Volatility: *Top note (page 16)*
Principal constitutents: *Cineole (70–80%), pinene*

Properties, effects, and methods of use

Essential oil of eucalyptus is a strong natural antiseptic that may be effective against a wide range of bacterial and viral infections. It has an overall cooling effect on the body and is useful in reducing fevers. The oil is clear with a strong camphoraceous smell that makes it a good insect repellant.

Emotional Uplifting and invigorating; clears and stimulates the mind and helps to prevent drowsiness. Used in inhalations, vaporizers, baths, application, or massage.

Respiratory Antiseptic and decongestant; helps to fight and prevent colds, flu, throat infections, sinusitis, and headaches caused by congestion; eases tight, dry coughs; relieves the breathlessness of asthma and bronchitis by loosening mucus. Used in gargles, inhalations, vaporizers, baths, application, or massage.

Skin Cooling and antiseptic; effective in the treatment of boils, pimples, head lice, and *herpes simplex*. Used in compresses or application.

Circulatory Cleansing; stimulates and is antiseptic to the urinary tract. Used in baths, massage, or application.

Muscular Anti-inflammatory; reduces swelling and helps to relieve muscular aches and pains, rheumatism, and arthritis. Used in compresses, baths, application, or massage.

Eucalyptus oil may also help to alleviate cystitis, when used in baths, application, or massage.

Caution: Once absorbed into the bloodstream, eucalyptus oil can irritate the kidneys if used in too high concentrations – keep to recommended dilutions.

Oils containing 1,8-cineole are regarded as toxic in Australia.

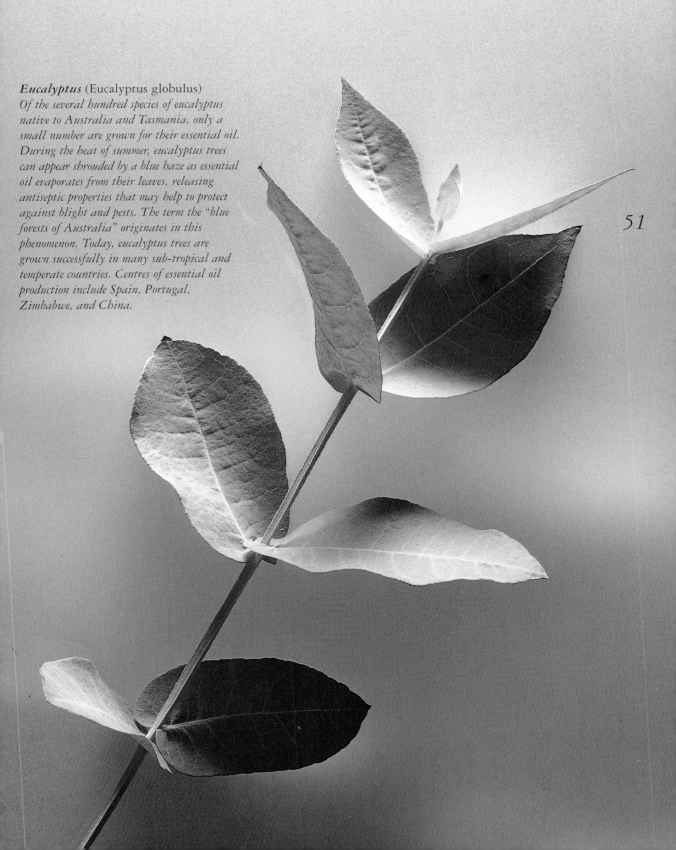

Eucalyptus (Eucalyptus globulus)
Of the several hundred species of eucalyptus
native to Australia and Tasmania, only a
small number are grown for their essential oil.
During the heat of summer, eucalyptus trees
can appear shrouded by a blue haze as essential
oil evaporates from their leaves, releasing
antiseptic properties that may help to protect
against blight and pests. The term the "blue
forests of Australia" originates in this
phenomenon. Today, eucalyptus trees are
grown successfully in many sub-tropical and
temperate countries. Centres of essential oil
production include Spain, Portugal,
Zimbabwe, and China.

Respiratory Problems

The respiratory tract has a thin, moist lining, the mucous membrane, which can become inflamed as a result of infection or allergic reaction. Swelling of the affected membrane narrows the nasal passages and makes breathing more difficult. Sometimes, secondary infections, such as sinusitis and bronchitis, may also develop. For both prevention and relief of respiratory problems, try to ensure that you have access to plenty of fresh air and avoid excessively dusty or smoky surroundings. Smokers must give up, or at least drastically cut down. Certain essential oils will help to reduce inflammation and loosen mucus; others have strong antiseptic properties that may help fight infection.

Throat Infection

A sore throat may be one of the first signs of a respiratory disorder, or it may develop in the secondary stages of an infection as a result of mucus being continually coughed up. Loss of voice (laryngitis) may also occur.

Useful Oils

Sandalwood, clary sage, and lavender are all soothing oils and excellent for a dry, sore throat, while the addition of such antiseptic oils as lemon, geranium, or tea tree may help to fight infection. Include eucalyptus, peppermint, and Atlas cedarwood where mucus is also present.

Treatment

Gargle Add *2 drops each of sandalwood and lemon* or *2 drops each of Atlas cedarwood and eucalyptus* to half a glass of water. At the onset of symptoms, gargle (page 21) with the mixture every few hours.

Application or Massage Dilute *3 drops of sandalwood, 2 drops of eucalyptus, and 1 drop of peppermint in ½fl oz (15ml/2½tsp) of lotion*, and apply the mixture to your face and chest. Or, ask a friend to give you a face and chest massage (pages 28 and 29), using the same blend mixed in oil rather than lotion.

Colds and Flu

The common cold is an infection of the upper respiratory tract characterized by soreness and inflammation of the nose and throat and mucus congestion. Influenza is a more serious viral infection, associated with fever, aching, and swollen lymph nodes. Aromatherapy treatment given in the early stages can help to prevent germs becoming established, but with the common cold, prevention is usually more effective than cure.

Useful Oils

Tea tree, lemon, geranium, and black pepper may help to combat infection. Lavender, rosemary, and, again, tea tree have a generalized beneficial effect and can give a boost to your immune system (page 35). Where the chest is affected, eucalyptus, peppermint, and Atlas cedarwood are all useful since they can loosen mucus.

Prevention

Diet To help prevent colds, include plenty of vitamin-C-rich foods (page 36) in your diet.

Gargle If there is flu in your area, gargle daily (page 21) with *1 drop each of tea tree and lemon* diluted in *½ a glass of water*. Stir well before each mouthful.

Treatment
Gargle At the onset of a cold or flu, gargle (page 21) with *2 drops each of tea tree and geranium.* Repeat every morning and night.
Inhalation If your head is heavy with a cold, add *1 drop each of peppermint, eucalyptus, and tea tree* to a bowl of hot water and inhale (page 21) every evening. **Caution:** Do not use this method if you have asthma (see opposite). To clear your head during the day, sprinkle *a few drops of lemon* on to a tissue and inhale.

Sinusitis

The most common forerunner of sinusitis is the common cold, but the condition may also be brought on by such diverse factors as foggy weather, tobacco smoke, excessive consumption of mucus-producing dairy products, and stress (page 36). It may also be induced by hay fever. Acute inflammation of the nasal passages can be very painful, causing headaches, and, sometimes, a blocked nose and earache as side effects.

Useful Oils
A combination of eucalyptus, peppermint, and lavender will help to clear nasal passages and relieve any accompanying headache.

Treatment
Inhalation Sprinkle *2 drops of eucalyptus and 1 drop each of peppermint and lavender* on to a tissue and inhale (page 21) deeply three times. Repeat every morning and night.
Application Spread the *Lotion* below thinly over your face every night, applying pressure as shown in illus b, page 31.

Anti-inflammatory and Decongestant Lotion
  2 drops of peppermint
  4 drops of eucalyptus
  3 drops of lavender
  ¹/₂fl oz (15ml/2¹/₂tsp) of carrier lotion

Dilute the essential oils in the lotion and use for application, as indicated.

Chronic Bronchitis and Asthma

Exposure to cigarette smoke and other external pollutants may cause irritation of the bronchial tubes, resulting in the excessive production of mucus and continual cough that characterize chronic bronchitis. Asthma may be brought on by similarly irritant substances, or it may occur in response to anxiety (page 44). **Caution:** Consult your doctor if an asthma attack is severe or if acute bronchitis develops, and is accompanied by a fever and painful cough.

Useful Oils
Atlas cedarwood, eucalyptus, and peppermint are decongestant oils that will help to clear air passages and loosen mucus; cajuput, pine, and tea tree also have a cleansing effect. Sweet marjoram and sandalwood can effectively soothe inflamed bronchi.

Treatment
Lifestyle Smokers must give up or cut down substantially for treatment to work.
Inhalation Sprinkle *a few drops each of cajuput, Atlas cedarwood, and eucalyptus* on to a tissue and inhale (page 21) deeply three times. Then place the tissue close to your chest. In an emergency, put *1 drop of cajuput* into your palm, cup your hands together and cover your nose. Inhale deeply. **Caution:** If you are asthmatic, do not inhale essential oils from a bowl of hot water, since concentrated steam can cause choking.
Application and Massage Dilute *3 drops of Atlas cedarwood, 2 drops of peppermint, and 1 drop of cajuput in ¹/₂fl oz (15ml/2¹/₂tsp) of carrier lotion,* and apply the mixture evenly to your chest and throat. You may also find it helpful to have your chest and upper back massaged (pages 29 and 25) with the same blend of essential oils mixed in ¹/₂fl oz (15ml/2¹/₂tsp) of *carrier oil.* Ask your friend to concentrate on moving his or her thumbs up the spinal column (illus b, page 25) since this will help to release and expel mucus.

Essential Oil of Rosemary

Part of plant used: *Flowering tops*
Method of extraction: *Steam distillation*
Volatility: *Middle note (page 16)*
Principal constituents: Cineole, *borneol, pinene*

Properties, effects, *and methods of use*

Essential oil of rosemary is noted for its strongly antiseptic and stimulating properties. It is also a gentle analgesic and regulator that helps to balance body and mind. It has a slightly camphoraceous, warm, pungent aroma.

Emotional Stimulating and astringent; stimulates the memory, clears the mind, and helps to relieve headaches, migraines, and general fatigue. Used in inhalations, vaporizers, baths, application, or massage.

Respiratory Antiseptic and antispasmodic; relieves coughs, colds, and flu. Used in inhalations, compresses, or massage.

Skin Cleansing and stimulating; effective against head lice; helps to prevent dandruff and hair loss, Used in rinses, application, or massage.

Digestive Antiseptic and gas/wind relieving; helps indigestion, flatulence, constipation, colitis, gastroenteritis, and stomach pains; also stimulates the liver. Used in compresses, application, or massage.

Circulatory Tonic and astringent; helps to raise blood pressure (a very low dose will lower it), improve circulation, and reduce lymphatic congestion; relieves fluid retention, cellulite, and varicose veins. Used in baths, application, or massage.

Muscular Gentle analgesic without sedative effects; relieves general aches and pains, sprains, and arthritis. Used in compresses, application, or massage.

Gynaecological Stimulating and normalizing; helps to regulate the menstrual cycle. Used in baths, application, or massage.

Caution: Avoid use during first five months of pregnancy (page v) or if you suffer from epilepsy.

Oils containing 1,8-cineole are regarded as toxic in Australia.

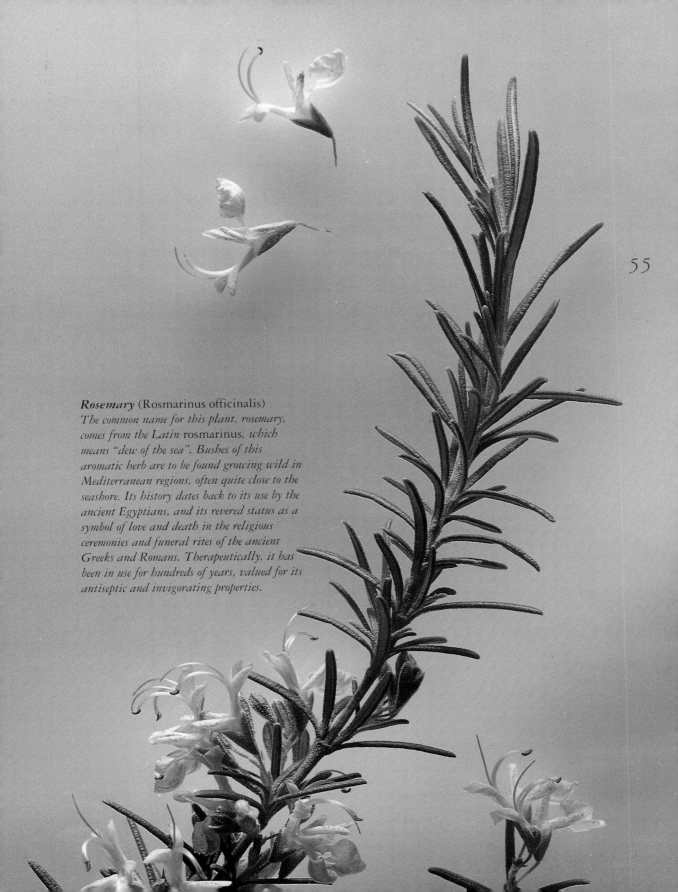

Rosemary (Rosmarinus officinalis)
The common name for this plant, rosemary,
comes from the Latin rosmarinus, *which*
means "dew of the sea". Bushes of this
aromatic herb are to be found growing wild in
Mediterranean regions, often quite close to the
seashore. Its history dates back to its use by the
ancient Egyptians, and its revered status as a
symbol of love and death in the religious
ceremonies and funeral rites of the ancient
Greeks and Romans. Therapeutically, it has
been in use for hundreds of years, valued for its
antiseptic and invigorating properties.

Skin and Hair Disorders

Skin forms the body's wall of defence against invading organisms, such as viruses and bacteria. It is covered in a mixture of sebum, an oily substance secreted by glands attached to the hair follicles, and sweat, which comes from the pores. For your skin to remain smooth and supple, sebum and sweat must be present in the correct proportions. A variety of factors, including too frequent washing, an unhealthy diet, hormonal imbalance, and stress (page 36), may affect the production of both substances, causing too much or too little to be secreted, with consequent greasy or dry skin. Many essential oils have normalizing properties and can play a major role in stabilizing the skin's acid balance.

Eczema

Eczema or dermatitis, as it is otherwise known, is a non-contagious skin disorder. Although there are various types, symptoms characteristically include itchy, dry, or weeping skin that may often be raw and painful, and sometimes bleed. Contact eczema (dermatitis) is a common form, which develops as an allergic reaction with itching, redness, and blistering occurring over those areas of skin that are exposed to the irritant. Atopic eczema affects people who have a family history of more generalized allergic reactions, such as asthma and hay fever, and is indicated by very dry, intensely itchy skin. In both cases, scratching may cause dry skin to crack and weep, and in some cases become infected. Stress (page 36) may aggravate symptoms so you should be prepared for your eczema to flare up if you are experiencing emotional problems.

Useful Oils

Roman chamomile and cypress help to relieve eczema because of their anti-inflammatory properties. Geranium and lavender are healing, while juniper berry helps to purify the blood. Sandalwood should be included where the skin is dry.

Treatment

If your eczema is part of an allergic reaction, you may need to adjust your diet or environment in order to identify the allergen. Begin by following the dietary guidelines given opposite under acne, seeking professional advice if need be.

Compress Make up a cold compress (page 21), cutting holes for the nose and eyes if it is for the face. Use a mixture of *2 drops each of Roman chamomile and lavender and 1 drop of geranium* and carefully apply the compress to the affected area.

Application or Massage If your skin is weeping and moist, add *4 drops each of lavender and geranium and 3 drops of juniper berry* to *1fl oz (30 ml/5tsp) of carrier lotion* and apply the mixture every morning and night to affected areas. For dry eczema, add *1 drop of sandalwood* to the above blend of essential oils and use carrier oil instead of lotion. Again, apply the mixture every morning and night. If your eczema is aggravated by stress, massage the lotion or oil mix into your shoulders and neck (page 31). Alternatively, you can ask a friend to use the oil mix to massage your back, shoulders, and neck (pages 25 and 24).

Acne

Acne usually results from hormonal imbalance or an incorrect diet, both being factors that affect the production of sebum. Stress (page 36) can also aggravate the condition. If secreted in excess of the skin's needs, sebum will build up in hair follicles and oily areas around the nose and chin. Spots and inflammation may occur where the sebum becomes trapped under the skin.

Useful Oils

Essential oils that regulate sebum production and purify the blood include juniper berry, lemon, and Atlas cedarwood. Lavender, cajuput, and geranium are antiseptic and healing, while Roman chamomile and petitgrain help to reduce inflammation.

Treatment

Lifestyle Gentle ultraviolet rays can greatly relieve acne so take every opportunity you can to go out in the sun, but be careful not to overexpose your skin.

Diet Eat a healthy, balanced diet, avoiding spicy and fatty foods, in particular dairy products. Include plenty of other sources of protein and calcium-rich sesame seeds. Drink up to four pints of spring water daily.

Application Add 5 *drops each of juniper berry and Atlas cedarwood* to a basin containing half a cup of distilled or spring water. Soak cotton balls/cotton wool pads in the mixture, then squeeze them gently and store them in a small plastic container. Wipe your skin with the balls/pads every two hours during the day, and use the mixture to bathe your skin at night. To complement this treatment, make up an oil mix by adding *3 drops each of lemon, petitgrain, and Atlas cedarwood* to *1fl oz (30ml/5tsp) of jojoba oil*. Then add the same blend of essential oils to *1fl oz (30ml/5tsp) of lotion*. Use the oil sparingly at night to cover your face and neck, and keep the lotion for morning application. Do not squeeze spots since this can cause inflammation and scarring.

Stretchmarks

When the skin is stretched over a long period of time, during pregnancy for example, it tends to lose some of its elasticity, and white or silvery purple stretchmarks may occur. The areas most likely to be affected in pregnancy are the lower abdomen and breasts; adolescent girls who have been overweight may get stretchmarks on their thighs and breasts. While it is not possible to return overstretched skin to its normal state, essential oils do have amazing regenerative powers and can help to improve the look of the skin. In pregnancy, prevention is better than cure, and with diligent use of oils stretchmarks need rarely occur.

Useful Oils

Regenerative oils such as lavender, frankincense, and myrrh are the best oils both for prevention and for minimizing existing stretchmarks. Geranium may be used in addition to help improve skin tone. The most effective carrier oil for relieving this condition is calendula. It is expensive, but you can mix it half and half with a sunflower or sweet almond vegetable base oil.

Prevention

Application To help keep the skin moist and supple and to prevent stretchmarks, apply the *Anti-stretchmark Oil* below every morning and night to susceptible areas, starting in the fourth month of pregnancy.

Treatment

Application Apply the *Anti-stretchmark Oil* below to affected areas every morning and night. Regular use is essential.

Anti-stretchmark Oil
> *3 drops each of frankincense and myrrh*
> *6 drops of lavender*
> *4 drops of geranium*
> *2fl oz (60ml/10tsp) of calendula carrier oil*

Add the essential oils to the carrier oil and use for application, as indicated.

The Ailments

Essential Oil of Geranium

Part of plant used: *Leaves*
Method of extraction: *Steam distillation*
Volatility: *Middle note (page 16)*
Principal constituents: *Geraniol, citronellol, linalol*

Properties, effects, and methods of use

Essential oil of geranium is a good all-rounder. It is effective in cleansing the body, and uplifting the mind. The oil has a rich, sweet aroma and is usually greenish-yellow in colour.

Emotional Uplifting; useful against stress; alleviates depression and anxiety. Used in inhalations, vaporizers, baths, application, or massage.

Respiratory Anti-infections; relieves throat and mouth infections. Used in mouthwashes or gargles.

Skin Astringent and balancing; cleanses and tones the skin; reduces inflammation; relieves acne, dry eczema, head lice, dandruff, *Herpes simplex*, stretchmarks and minor wounds; soothes measles' rashes in children. Used in baths, compresses, or application.

Digestive Tonic and cleansing; stimulates the liver; effective against mouth ulcers, diarrhoea, and gastroenteritis. Used in compresses, baths, application, or massage.

Circulatory Astringent, stimulant, and antiseptic; assists elimination of waste products; can help to relieve fluid retention and cellulite. Used in baths, application, or massage.

Gynaecological Stimulant and regulator of hormone production; helpful for pre-menstrual syndrome, menopausal symptoms, vaginal infections, and sterility. Used in inhalations, compresses, baths, application, or massage.

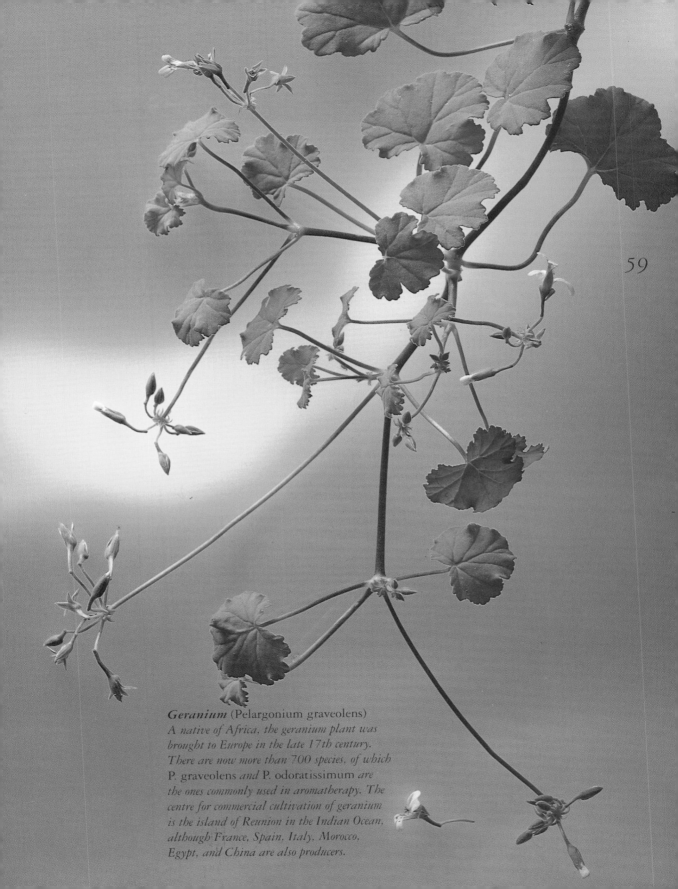

Geranium (Pelargonium graveolens)
A native of Africa, the geranium plant was
brought to Europe in the late 17th century.
There are now more than 700 species, of which
P. graveolens *and* P. odoratissimum *are*
the ones commonly used in aromatherapy. The
centre for commercial cultivation of geranium
is the island of Reunion in the Indian Ocean,
although France, Spain, Italy, Morocco,
Egypt, and China are also producers.

Herpes Simplex

The virus *Herpes simplex* I manifests itself as blisters around the mouth; a second strain, *Herpes simplex II*, produces similar symptoms in the genital area and can be sexually transmitted. The common cold, exhaustion, and general poor health may all serve to activate the herpes virus, which is always present in our bodies. In the first type, the blisters burst open to form "cold sores". If untreated, these may persist and spread to a larger area before the virus dies.

Caution: If symptoms persist, seek medical advice. *Herpes simplex I* can be transferred to the eyes, causing dendritic ulcers, so be sure to keep your fingers away from your eyes and to change your washcloth/face cloth and towel daily, using them to clean and dry the eye area first. If the virus gets into your eyes, you should consult an ophthalmic optician immediately.

Useful Oils

Geranium and lemon are thought to have anti-viral powers, while eucalyptus or lavender have antiseptic properties that may be useful. A treatment combining these oils can help to relieve symptoms.

Treatment

Application Add *4 drops each of lemon, eucalyptus, and geranium to ¹/₂fl oz (15ml/2¹/₂tsp) of lotion or calendula carrier oil*. Transfer the mixture to a brown glass bottle and apply regularly to affected areas.

Athlete's Foot

Thickened, moist skin between the toes is the first sign of athlete's foot, a condition caused by a fungal growth, *Tinea pedis*. Later the skin becomes itchy and dries before cracking and peeling off.

Useful Oils

Tagetes, lavender, and tea tree have anti-fungal powers that may help this condition.

Treatment

Lifestyle Dry your feet thoroughly after washing, particularly between the toes, and change socks or tights frequently.

Footbath Soak your feet for ten minutes every evening in a bowl of warm water to which you have added *2 drops each of tagetes, lavender, and tea tree*. Dry your feet thoroughly after soaking them.

Compress As an alternative to a footbath, apply a warm compress (page 21) to your foot, using the same blend of oils. Cover the compress with plastic wrap/cling film and wear a sock to keep it in place overnight.

Application Add the same blend of oils to ¹/₂fl oz (15ml/2¹/₂tsp) of calendula carrier oil and apply the mix evenly between your toes. Repeat every morning, using the footbath or compress treatment last thing at night before you go to bed.

Dandruff

Dandruff may take the form of fine, dry, powdery flakes or coarse, waxy scales that stick to the hair and scalp, causing intense irritation. With the latter type of dandruff, resist the temptation to scratch your head since this may cause bleeding and infection. If your facial skin becomes oily and pimples/spots develop, wash your hair frequently and choose a hairstyle that keeps hair off the forehead. This condition can easily be confused with either eczema (page 56) or psoriasis of the scalp, so it is important to obtain an accurate diagnosis from a trichologist (scalp and hair specialist).

Useful Oils

For greasy dandruff, use antiseptic and balancing oils such as juniper berry, Atlas cedarwood, rosemary, and lemon. Very dry, flaky scalps and dry hair are best treated with soothing oils such as lavender, geranium, and sandalwood.

Skin and Hair Disorders

Treatment

Lifestyle and Diet If you are prone to oily, scaling dandruff, wash your hair frequently, using a mild shampoo. Take plenty of exercise outdoors in the fresh air and follow the dietary advice given under acne on page 57. Dry dandruff is often stress-related. To prevent a build-up of tension, follow the anti-stress measures recommended on page 36.

Application Choose one of the recipes below and apply it to your scalp, leaving for two hours or overnight. Shampoo and rinse thoroughly. Make up a final rinse by adding the same blend of essential oils to a jug of water. Stir well before applying. Repeat the treatment every one or two days, decreasing to twice a week if symptoms begin to improve. If your scalp becomes red and itchy, try the following treatment. Add *2 drops each of geranium and lavender, 3 drops of juniper berry, and 1 drop of sandalwood to ½fl oz (15ml/ 2½tsp) of carrier lotion or oil.* Apply a small amount of the mixture to inflamed areas and leave it overnight, washing the hair with a mild, unperfumed shampoo the next morning. Repeat the treatment every two or three days. If your symptoms fail to improve, you should seek the advice of a trichologist (scalp and hair specialist).

Oil for a Dry, Flaking Scalp
 5 drops of lavender
 5 drops of geranium
 2 drops of sandalwood
 1fl oz (30ml/5tsp) of carrier oil

Lotion for an Oily, Scaling Scalp
 6 drops of Atlas cedarwood
 4 drops of rosemary
 4 drops of lemon
 1fl oz (30ml/5tsp) of carrier lotion

Choose whichever recipe corresponds to your type of dandruff. Mix the essential oils with the carrier and use for application, as indicated.

Hair Loss

Temporary hair loss may be part of a reaction to extreme stress or a sudden shock, or it may occur after giving birth, following a serious illness, or as a side effect of drug treatment. It can also be part of an allergic response. Stress-related tension in particular, can tighten the scalp and hinder nutrient-rich blood from reaching the hair follicles. As a result, the food-starved roots shrink within the follicles and hair may start to be lost. Male pattern baldness affects selected areas of the scalp; it is linked to hereditary factors but may be triggered by lifestyle or diet. **Caution:** Patchy baldness may indicate ringworm or another skin condition and should be referred to a trichologist (scalp and hair specialist) for an accurate diagnosis.

Useful Oils
Rosemary and ylang ylang will stimulate the scalp, while lavender and Atlas cedarwood are balancing oils that help to prevent further hair loss.

Treatment
Massage Gentle nightly massage of the scalp will relieve any tightness caused by stress. Make up the *Healthy Scalp Tonic* below and apply several drops to the affected area. Massage in such a way that you move the scalp over the bone without pulling, or moving through, the hair. Continue for two minutes, moving on to a different area every 15 seconds. Alternatively, ask a friend to give you a regular scalp massage (page 28).

Healthy Scalp Tonic
 3 drops each of rosemary and ylang ylang
 2 drops of Atlas cedarwood
 ½tsp of vodka
 1fl oz (30ml/5tsp) of orange flower or melissa water

Dissolve the essential oils in the vodka, then mix together with the orange flower or melissa water. Use for massage, as indicated.

Essential Oil of Peppermint

Part of plant used: *Leaves*
Method of extraction: *Steam distillation*
Volatility: *Middle note (page 16)*
Principal constituents: *Menthol, limonene, menthone*

Properties, effects, and methods of use

Essential oil of peppermint promotes overall physical and emotional wellbeing, although its healing properties are primarily associated with the digestive system. It has a light, clean, refreshing aroma, and is a good insect repellant.

Emotional Stimulating and strengthening; uplifts the system and is especially useful in the treatment of shock; helpful for neuralgia and relief of general debility, headaches, and migraines. Used in inhalations, baths, or application.

Respiratory Antiseptic and antispasmodic; effective in reducing mucus and relieving coughs, sinusitis, throat infections, colds, flu, asthma, and bronchitis. Used in inhalations, baths, or application.

Skin Cooling and cleansing; soothes itchy skin (see caution below); relieves inflammation and congestion. Used in baths or application.

Digestive Soothing and antispasmodic; relieves acidity, heartburn, diarrhoea, indigestion, and flatulence; also highly effective for travel sickness and nausea; helps to combat bad breath. Used in gargles or application.

Circulatory Cooling; helpful for varicose veins and haemorrhoids. Used in compresses or application.

Gynaecological Cooling and decongestant; encourages menstrual regularity; relieves hot flashes/flushes. Used in baths, application, or massage.

Caution: Too concentrated a dose of peppermint oil can cause itchiness – keep to recommended dilutions. Keep your eyes closed when inhaling.

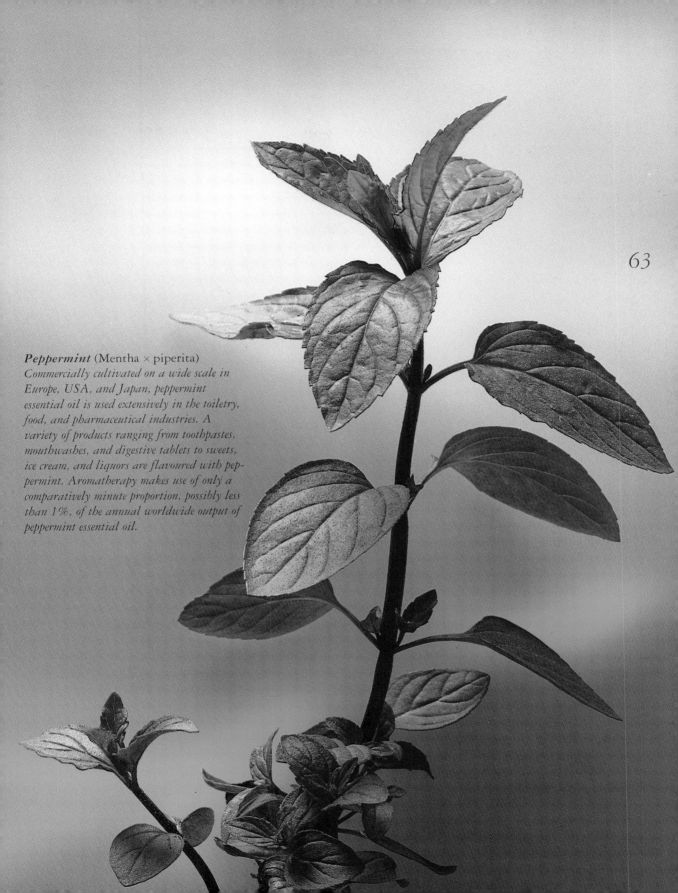

Peppermint (Mentha × piperita)
*Commercially cultivated on a wide scale in
Europe, USA, and Japan, peppermint
essential oil is used extensively in the toiletry,
food, and pharmaceutical industries. A
variety of products ranging from toothpastes,
mouthwashes, and digestive tablets to sweets,
ice cream, and liquors are flavoured with peppermint. Aromatherapy makes use of only a
comparatively minute proportion, possibly less
than 1%, of the annual worldwide output of
peppermint essential oil.*

Digestive Problems

The normal functioning of the digestive system can easily be disrupted by poor eating habits. A natural wholefood diet including plenty of fibre and liquid (page 36), and regular meals will help to keep stools firm but moist and facilitate their passage out of the body. In addition, many essential oils can, through their stimulant, astringent, or antispasmodic properties, help to maintain or restore the healthy functioning of your digestive system. Used in inhalations, application, or massage, they may be as effective in relieving digestive problems as when taken internally; the latter form of treatment is *not* recommended for self-help (see list of Points to Observe on page 19).

Heartburn

Heartburn is a form of indigestion character-ized by a tight, burning sensation in the mid-dle of the chest. The unpleasant taste that often accompanies it is caused by gastric acid flowing up from the stomach. This condition may stem from over-hasty eating, an unfortu-nate combination of foods, or an emotional reaction. In pregnant (see cautions on page v) and overweight women, increased pressure on the stomach may give rise to heartburn.

Useful Oils
Peppermint and lemon are digestive oils, while sandalwood encourages relaxation.

Treatment
Massage Apply a little of the *Lotion* below to your breastbone and the area just beneath. Use the palm of your hand and massage in a clockwise, circular motion, applying firm pressure.

Acidity-regulating Lotion
    2 drops each of lemon and peppermint
    3 drops of sandalwood
    ¹/₂fl oz (15ml/2¹/₂tsp) of carrier lotion

Mix the essential oils with the carrier lotion and use for massage, as indicated.

Indigestion and Flatulence

Frequent bouts of indigestion or flatulence are often a result of poor dietary habits, including overeating, eating too quickly, and going for long periods without food. You may also experience discomfort if you eat a meal when emotionally tense. **Caution:** If your indigestion progressively worsens or is associated with weight loss, consult your doc-tor since either may indicate a more serious problem, such as a peptic ulcer or gallstone.

Useful Oils
Lemon, caraway, peppermint, ginger, juniper berry, lavender, rosemary, Roman chamomile, and sweet marjoram all assist the digestion.

Treatment
Diet Avoid gas-inducing foods, such as peas and beans, and carbonated beverages.
Application or Massage Add *4 drops of peppermint and 2 drops each of juniper berry and caraway to ¹/₂fl oz (15ml/¹/₂tsp) of lotion.* Apply the mixture to your upper or lower abdomen, depending on where you feel the discomfort. Or, ask a friend to use the same mix to massage the upper or lower area of your abdomen (page 30).

Mouth Ulcers

Mouth ulcers may be due to poor diet, vitamin deficiency, stomach or intestinal upsets, or food allergy. They usually appear on the lining of the gums and cheek, or along the edge of the tongue, and are more likely to erupt if you are under stress (page 36) or exhausted from lack of sleep or overwork. Ulcers may also appear in the mouth as a result of a bacterial, viral, or fungal infection; these types of ulcer can be most effectively treated with aromatherapy. **Caution:** Consult your doctor if you have painless or persistent mouth ulcers, or if they arise in white patches, or are coexistent with genital sores.

Useful Oils

Highly antiseptic oils, such as tea tree, lemon, and geranium, may work well on ulcers of viral or bacterial origin. Myrrh, tea tree, and lavender are thought to have useful antifungal properties.

Treatment

Diet Eat a healthy, balanced diet (page 36), including foods that are rich in B vitamins.
Application Mix *5 drops of tea tree, 3 drops of lemon, and 2 drops of myrrh with ½fl oz (15ml/ 2½tsp) of carrier oil* and apply with your finger to ulcerated areas at regular intervals throughout the day.
Mouthwash In addition, add *1 drop each of tea tree, geranium, and lavender to ½ a glass of water* and use three or four times a day as a mouthwash (page 21).

Diarrhoea

Consumption of food that is infected with bacteria is a common cause of diarrhoea. It may also result from a viral infection, an intolerance to certain foods or drugs, a change in diet, or intense emotions such as anxiety or fear. On-going stress (page 36) can also disrupt the digestive process, causing a chronic form of this condition to develop.

Caution: Acute attacks of diarrhoea accompanied by severe vomiting may indicate serious food poisoning and medical help should be sought. Consult your doctor also if an attack persists for more than a couple of days or keeps recurring.

Useful Oils

Drying, astringent oils include cypress, juniper berry, geranium, and lemon, while sandalwood is soothing. Peppermint and Roman chamomile are good antispasmodics, while tea tree has useful bactericidal properties. Sandalwood, Roman chamomile, and geranium are also relaxing oils and therefore can be helpful where stress is known to be a contributory factor.

Prevention

When travelling in hot countries, take care to peel all fruit and salad vegetables and to drink only bottled water.

Treatment

Diet To prevent dehydration during an attack, make up a drink using the juice of a fresh orange, half a teaspoonful of salt, and 1 teaspoonful of honey. Fill the glass up to the top with water and sip continually until symptoms improve.
Massage Use the *Astringent and Stabilizing Mix* below to massage your lower abdomen and the small of your back (page 32), working in a clockwise direction. Repeat every few hours until symptoms improve. Alternatively, ask a friend to massage these areas for you (pages 30 and 25).
Bath Sprinkle *3 drops each of geranium and juniper berry and 2 drops of peppermint* into your bath water.

Astringent and Stabilizing Mix
   3 drops each of tea tree and peppermint
   2 drops each of geranium and sandalwood
   1fl oz (30ml/5tsp) of carrier lotion or oil

Mix the essential oils with the carrier lotion or oil and use for massage, as indicated.

65

Essential Oil of Cypress

Part of plant used: *Twigs, needles, and cones*
Method of extraction: *Steam distillation*
Volatility: *Middle note (page 16)*
Principal constituents: *Pinene, carene, cedrol*

Properties, effects, and methods of use

Essential oil of cypress is primarily beneficial to the circulatory and vascular systems. It also has both astringent and styptic properties (the latter causes constriction of blood vessels and helps to staunch blood loss). The oil is slightly yellow in colour and has a rich, woody aroma.

Emotional Sedative and soothing; helps to clear the mind of grief and prepare it for sleep; useful against insomnia. Used in inhalations, vaporizers, baths, application, or massage.

Respiratory Antispasmodic and antiseptic; relieves asthma, spasmodic coughs, and laryngitis. Used in gargles, inhalations, vaporizers, baths, or application.

Skin Astringent and soothing; may help to regulate production of sebum in greasy skin; reduces sweating; can relieve eczema. Used in application.

Digestive Antiseptic and antispasmodic; soothes attacks of diarrhoea. Used in baths or application.

Circulatory Astringent and styptic; relieves fluid retention and cellulite; invaluable in the treatment of varicose veins, haemorrhoids, circulatory cramps, chilblains, and broken capillaries. Used in application.

Muscular Tonic; helpful for cramps; reduces swelling in rheumatism. Used in baths, compresses, application, or massage.

Gynaecological Antispasmodic and styptic; can help to staunch a haemorrhage or excessive blood loss; relieves painful menstruation and menopausal spotting; useful after childbirth as a means of controlling the amount of blood lost and for calming vulval tissues. Used in compresses, baths, application, or massage.

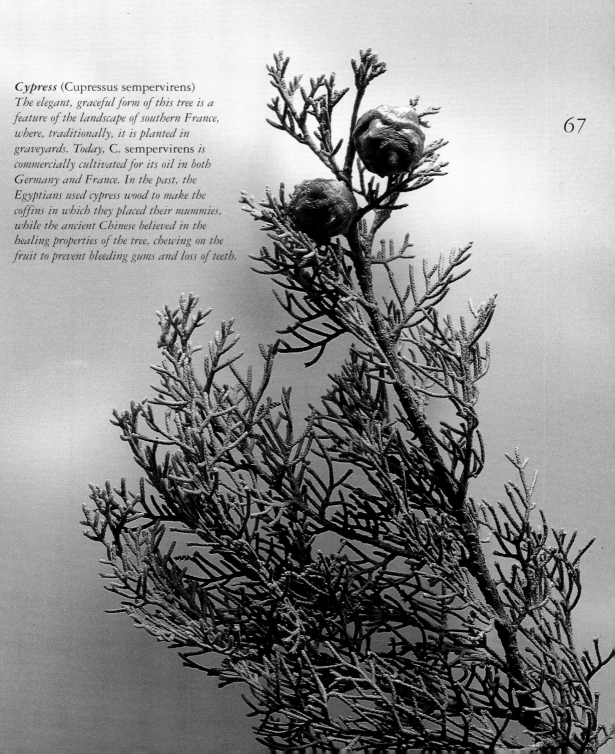

Cypress (Cupressus sempervirens)
The elegant, graceful form of this tree is a
feature of the landscape of southern France,
where, traditionally, it is planted in
graveyards. Today, C. sempervirens *is*
commercially cultivated for its oil in both
Germany and France. In the past, the
Egyptians used cypress wood to make the
coffins in which they placed their mummies,
while the ancient Chinese believed in the
healing properties of the tree, chewing on the
fruit to prevent bleeding gums and loss of teeth.

Nausea

Feelings of nausea do sometimes precede vomiting, but they also often occur independently. Heavy or fatty meals, obnoxious tastes or smells, and emotional stress may all give rise to nausea. It is also common during air, sea, and land travel, and during the early months of pregnancy (see cautions on page v) when women may experience it as "morning sickness".

Useful Oils

Emotional nausea is most likely to respond to relaxing oils such as sandalwood, lavender, and rose otto, while peppermint and black pepper will help to relieve symptoms associated with unhealthy eating habits. Include mandarin for morning sickness; for travel sickness, try caraway, ginger, and peppermint since these are settling to the stomach. Caraway and true melissa will help with any accompanying dizziness. If success is not achieved first time round, include one oil for each type of nausea, for example, lavender, peppermint, and ginger.

Prevention

Application To prevent travel sickness, add *4 drops of peppermint and 4 drops of caraway or ginger to 1fl oz (30ml/5tsp) of lotion or carrier oil.* Apply the mixture thinly to your chest and stomach before setting out on the journey. Use the same blend, minus the carrier, for inhaling during the trip, if necessary.

Treatment

Inhalation This method may be used effectively to relieve all types of nausea. Sprinkle *a few drops each of peppermint and lavender* on to a tissue, and add a few more drops of any one of the other oils that may be helpful for your type of nausea. Inhale deeply three times.

Application or Massage For food-related nausea, mix *3 drops each of peppermint and black pepper and 2 drops of rose otto* with *1fl oz (30ml/5tsp) of carrier lotion.* Apply the mix to your abdomen or ask a friend to massage that area for you (page 30).

Constipation

Constipation may result from insufficient exercise, lack of fibre in the diet, drug treatment, or simply a disruption of your habitual daily routine. It may also occur if you are exposed to on-going stress (page 36).

Caution: In an elderly person with previously normal bowel habits, constipation may be a sign of a more serious underlying disorder and should be referred to a doctor.

Useful oils

Roman chamomile, bitter orange, black pepper, mandarin, and rosemary stimulate the digestion and are the most effective oils for treating this condition. Where stress is a contributory factor, sweet marjoram and, again, Roman chamomile are helpful.

Treatment

Lifestyle Make a positive attempt to establish a regular time for defecating, for example, first thing in the morning after a hot drink. Take regular exercise: this is particularly important if you have a sedentary occupation.

Diet Try to drink plenty of fluids and eat natural wholefoods containing plenty of fibre, in particular fresh, unpeeled fruit and vegetables, and whole-grain cereals. Avoid regular use of herbal or chemical laxatives. These may be effective at first but they eventually weaken the muscles of the digestive tract and can cause chronic constipation.

Massage Regular self-massage is effective for this condition but should be complemented by the lifestyle and dietary advice given above. Make up a massage oil by adding *3 drops each of sweet marjoram and rosemary and 2 drops of Roman chamomile to 1fl oz (30ml/5tsp) of carrier oil.* Using firm but gentle strokes and working in a clockwise direction, massage the oil into your lower abdomen and the small of your back (page 32) for several minutes every day. Alternatively, ask a friend to massage these areas (pages 30 and 25) for you so you can relax more fully.

Circulatory Problems

The efficient circulation of blood and lymph is vital to health. Blood nourishes the body, transporting nutrients and oxygen to individual cells. Lymph removes excess fluid and toxic waste from our tissues. Both contain the white blood cells that enable us to fight and, in most cases, overcome invasion by foreign bodies, such as viruses and bacteria. Unhealthy eating habits, lack of exercise, and stress (page 36) can all adversely affect circulation and lower the immune response. Essential oils can pass directly into the bloodstream via the capillary walls. Some may help to stimulate and improve circulation, while others can effectively reduce high blood pressure.

Palpitations

Your heart may flutter or beat more forcefully or rapidly in response to emotions such as anger, fear, or excitement, following exercise, or after ingestion of stimulant drinks, certain drugs, or nicotine. Soothing essential oils can bring speedy relief, but if palpitations persist or are recurrent, you should seek medical advice.

Useful Oils

If the cause is emotional, calming oils such as neroli, true melissa, lavender, mandarin, and ylang ylang will help.

Treatment

Diet Avoid coffee, tea, and other caffeinated soft drinks. Smokers should give up, or cut down substantially.

Inhalation Place *1 drop of neroli* on your palm and cup your hands over your nose. Inhale deeply (page 21). Alternatively, sprinkle *a few drops each of neroli, lavender, and ylang ylang* on to a tissue, and inhale deeply.

Massage Ask a friend to massage your neck, chest, and back (pages 24, 29, and 25), using a mix made from *4 drops of neroli and 3 drops each of lavender and ylang ylang* diluted in *½fl oz (15ml/2½tsp) of carrier oil*.

Low Blood Pressure

Low blood pressure is physiological in a small number of people. It is generally considered to be healthy, but when accompanied by poor circulation, dizzy spells, and/or fainting, you should obtain an accurate diagnosis. These symptoms may result from a temporary fall in pressure, in which case they will respond well to aromatherapy. **Caution:** They can also indicate that the heart is failing, a condition that requires urgent medical attention. Over-medication for high blood pressure may give rise to similar symptoms.

Useful Oils

Invigorating oils such as black pepper and rosemary will help to improve circulation.

Treatment

Lifestyle Take regular exercise.

Massage Ask a friend to give you a regular body massage (pages 24 to 30), using a mix made by adding *3 drops each of rosemary and black pepper to ½fl oz (15ml/2½tsp) of carrier oil*. Alternatively, add the same essential oils to *½fl oz (15ml/2½tsp) of carrier lotion* and use the mix for self-massage (pages 31 to 32).

Bath For a stimulating bath, add *3 drops each of rosemary and black pepper* to the water.

Essential Oil of Juniper Berry

Part of plant used: *Ripe berries*
Method of extraction: *Steam distillation*
Volatility: *Middle note (page 16)*
Principal constituents: *Pinene, terpineol, cadinene*

Properties, effects, and methods of use

Essential oil of juniper berry is noted primarily for its antiseptic and diuretic properties. The oil is colourless to pale yellow when freshly distilled, but it grows darker and thicker with age. The fresh aroma is similar to that of cypress (both plants are from the same family), but sharper and more peppery.

Emotional Calming and a tonic; helpful in overcoming anxiety, insomnia, and mental fatigue. Used in baths, vaporizers, application, or massage.

Skin Astringent and cleansing; beneficial for acne, oily skin, greasy hair, dandruff, and weeping eczema. Used in masks, compresses, or application.

Digestive Antiseptic and purifying; relieves indigestion, flatulence, diarrhoea, and colic. Used in baths, compresses, application, or massage.

Circulatory Stimulant and diuretic; helps to lower blood pressure; cleanses the body, relieving fluid retention, cellulite, varicose veins, and haemorrhoids; stimulates the kidneys. Used in baths, application, or massage.

Muscular Analgesic; useful for muscular aches and pains and rheumatism. Used in compresses, baths, application, or massage.

Gynaecological Diuretic; can be helpful for irregular or painful menstruation; invaluable (with cypress) when breasts are swollen during menstruation. Alleviates fluid retention by assisting elimination of waste products. Used in compresses, baths, or application.

Juniper berry oil may also alleviate cystitis, when used in baths or application.

Caution: Avoid use during first five months of pregnancy (page v), and in cases of severe kidney disease where, once absorbed into the bloodstream, the oil can overstimulate the kidneys.

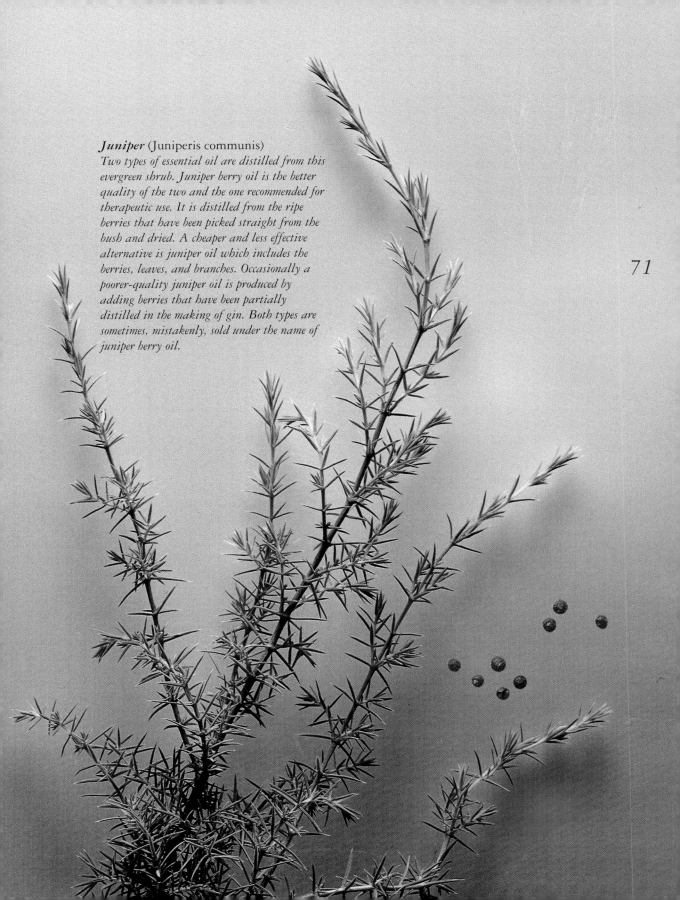

Juniper (Juniperis communis)
*Two types of essential oil are distilled from this
evergreen shrub. Juniper berry oil is the better
quality of the two and the one recommended for
therapeutic use. It is distilled from the ripe
berries that have been picked straight from the
bush and dried. A cheaper and less effective
alternative is juniper oil which includes the
berries, leaves, and branches. Occasionally a
poorer-quality juniper oil is produced by
adding berries that have been partially
distilled in the making of gin. Both types are
sometimes, mistakenly, sold under the name of
juniper berry oil.*

71

High Blood Pressure

The pressure at which the heart pumps blood through the body may differ slightly from person to person. It may also vary throughout the day, rising after physical exertion or in response to stress. When blood pressure remains raised over a prolonged period, resulting in hypertension, it may not necessarily be accompanied by other symptoms. For this reason, it is advisable to have your blood pressure checked at regular intervals by your doctor. A variety of lifestyle factors, including exposure to a high level of stress (page 36), smoking, and overconsumption of salt, alcohol, and fatty foods, may all indirectly lead to high blood pressure. **Caution:** Do not stop taking medication that your doctor has prescribed for you.

Useful Oils

Clary sage, lemon, sweet marjoram, true melissa, mandarin, and ylang ylang can all help to reduce pressure, while lavender encourages relaxation. Juniper berry can improve kidney function.

Treatment

If you can, visit a professional aromatherapist regularly for a full massage.

Lifestyle Take regular exercise, but avoid sudden or strenuous physical effort. Smokers should try to give up or cut down, using oils to combat stress if need be.

Diet Eat a healthy, balanced diet (page 36), reducing your intake of salt, sugar, animal fats, alcohol, and stimulant drinks. Garlic is particularly effective for lowering blood pressure and may be taken in capsule form. Alternatively, eat fresh, raw garlic and parsley in abundance.

Application Add the essential oils from the recipe below to ¹⁄₂fl oz (15ml/2¹⁄₂tsp) of carrier lotion. Apply the lotion to your chest and the soles of your feet every night.

Bath Add *3 drops each of sweet marjoram and ylang ylang* to an evening bath twice a week.

Massage Ask a friend to use the *Oil* below to massage your chest, abdomen, and back (pages 29, 30, and 25) on a regular basis.

Soothing Massage Oil
> *2 drops each of juniper berry and clary sage*
> *4 drops of lemon*
> *1 drop of ylang ylang*
> *¹⁄₂fl oz (15ml/2¹⁄₂tsp) of carrier oil*

Mix the essential oils with the carrier oil and use for massage, as indicated.

Fluid Retention

Prior to the onset of menstruation, fluid may build up in the abdomen and breasts. Retention of fluid may also occur in pregnancy (see cautions on page v), showing as "puffiness" on the legs and ankles. **Caution:** If symptoms persist, or in the case of more generalized swelling which may be linked to kidney or cardiac malfunction, you should seek the advice of your doctor.

Useful Oils

Juniper berry, lavender, and rosemary are all excellent diuretics; the first two will also help to reduce any accompanying stress (page 36). Geranium and cypress are both useful tonics.

Treatment

Massage Mix *3 drops of juniper berry and 2 drops each of rosemary and lavender* with 1fl oz (30ml/5tsp) of carrier oil. Ask a friend to use the mix to massage up the back of your legs and over your lower back and abdomen (pages 26, 25, and 30). For pre-menstrual fluid retention, begin treatment several days before you expect the swelling to show.

Compress To relieve pre-menstrual swelling, make up a warm compress (page 21) using *3 drops each of rosemary and juniper berry and 2 drops each of lavender and cypress.* Place over your abdomen and breasts every night for a week prior to menstruation.

Cellulite

This condition affects mainly women and shows as lumpy, puckered tissue, resembling orange peel, on the thighs, buttocks, and, sometimes, arms. It usually, but not always, occurs in overweight women, and is thought to be caused by a build-up of fluid and toxic waste products in the tissues due to poor lymphatic circulation. It is not to be confused with cellulitis, the medical term for inflammation of tissues through infection. Regular massage with essential oils will help to break down the lumps so that the fluid and toxins are reabsorbed into the lymphatic system and eliminated from the body.

Useful Oils

Juniper berry and geranium are detoxifying, and, together with the cleansing properties of rosemary, will help to reduce fluid. Decongestant oils include lavender and patchouli; cypress is a good tonic for the circulation.

Treatment

Massage Dilute *4 drops each of juniper berry and rosemary and 3 drops each of cypress and patchouli in 1fl oz (30ml/5tsp) of carrier oil or lotion.* Massage twice daily into affected areas, applying firm pressure with the palm of your hand and working in a circular motion. In addition, ask a friend to give you a daily back and leg massage (pages 25 and 26 to 27).

Varicose Veins

The flow of blood from the legs back up to the heart is assisted by muscular contractions and by valves that are sited in the veins so as to prevent backward flow. Standing or sitting for long periods, lack of exercise, and weakness in the valves themselves, can hinder the flow, causing blood to accumulate and the walls of the veins to become stretched. As a result, enlarged, twisted, blue veins, known as varicose veins, may appear on the legs; these are often quite painful.

Haemorrhoids are a type of varicose vein occurring in the rectum (internal piles) and around the anus (external piles). They may bleed during a bowel movement. Haemorrhoids that bleed persistently can cause anaemia and should be referred to a doctor. Constipation and abdominal pressure in pregnancy are two common causes.

Useful Oils

Peppermint, lemon, and cypress are astringent oils that encourage the veins to constrict. Lemon, juniper berry, and rosemary will stimulate circulation, while peppermint or sandalwood can soothe any irritation.

Treatment

Injection or removal of severe varicose veins is sometimes advised but this may be only a temporary solution since other veins are put under strain and the problem may recur. It is as well to consider other alternatives.

Lifestyle To reduce varicose veins in the legs, take regular walks. If you have to stand for long periods, raise your heels and toes frequently to contract your calf muscles.

Diet Reduce your meat and salt intake and eat plenty of parsley and garlic. To prevent recurrence of haemorrhoids, follow the dietary advice under constipation (page 68).

Application For relief of both varicose veins and haemorrhoids, use *3 drops of cypress, 2 drops of sandalwood, and 1 drop of peppermint* in *1fl oz (30ml/5tsp) of calendula carrier oil or lotion.* Apply to affected areas every morning and evening. **Caution**: Use your palms not your fingertips, and work from ankle toward the heart in an upward direction only.

Compress To relieve varicose veins, make up a cold compress (page 21) using *3 drops each of cypress and rosemary and 2 drops of peppermint.* Fix the compress securely in position, covering it first with plastic wrap/cling film. **Caution**: Never take hot baths – these increase the blood flow and can further stretch the venous walls.

Essential Oil of Sweet Marjoram

Part of plant used: *Leaves and flowering heads*
Method of extraction: *Steam distillation*
Volatility: *Middle note (page 16)*
Principal constituents: *Terpinen-4-ol, pinene*

Properties, effects, and methods of use

Sweet marjoram essential oil has profoundly warming properties that are soothing and comforting to both body and mind. The oil has a mild, light aroma that is pleasing if you are in low spirits.

Emotional Calming and sedative; helpful in the relief of anxiety and tension, general debility, insomnia, irritability, and hysteria; can provide comfort for those suffering from intangible emotions such as grief, loneliness, and rejection; relieves headaches and migraines. Used in inhalations, vaporizers, baths, application, or massage.

Respiratory Soothing and warming; alleviates bronchitis and asthma. Used in inhalations, vaporizers, compresses, baths, application, or massage.

Circulatory Calming; can help to lower high blood pressure. Used in inhalations, vaporizers, compresses, baths, application, or massage.

Digestive Antispasmodic and soothing; helps to relieve constipation, indigestion, flatulence, and colic. Used in application or massage.

Muscular Warming and analgesic; relieves muscular cramps, spasms, aches and pains, neuralgia, sprains, strains, rheumatism, and arthritis. Used in compresses, baths, application, or massage.

Gynaecological Antispasmodic; effective for menstrual pain. Calms sexual desire. Used in compresses, baths, application, or massage.

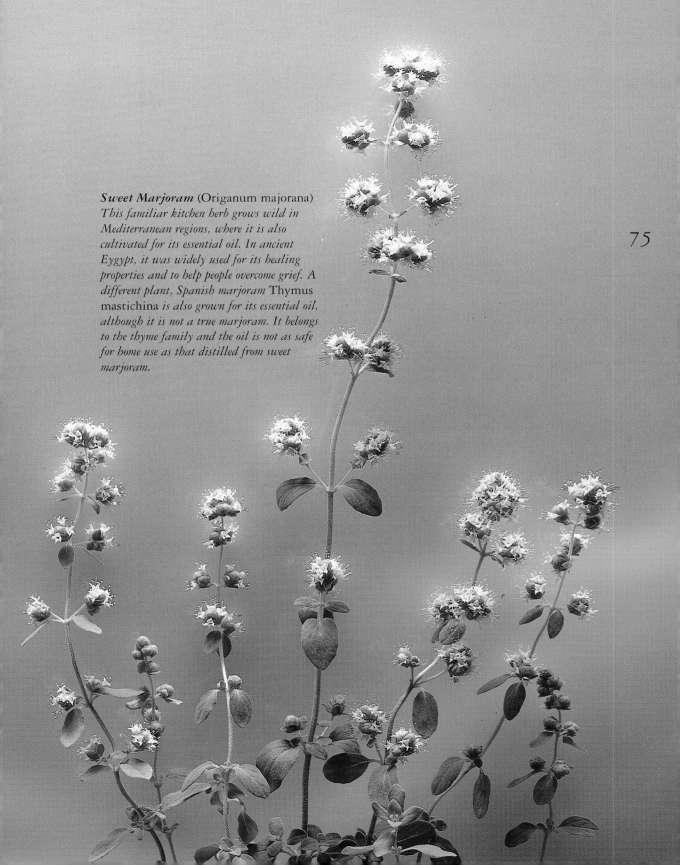

Sweet Marjoram (Origanum majorana)
This familiar kitchen herb grows wild in Mediterranean regions, where it is also cultivated for its essential oil. In ancient Eygypt, it was widely used for its healing properties and to help people overcome grief. A different plant, Spanish marjoram Thymus mastichina *is also grown for its essential oil, although it is not a true marjoram. It belongs to the thyme family and the oil is not as safe for home use as that distilled from sweet marjoram.*

75

Muscular Problems

The bony framework of the skeleton is covered by voluntary muscles that we can contract or relax at will. In contrast, the involuntary muscles of the heart and digestive system are outside of our immediate control. A healthy, balanced diet (page 36) will help to maintain healthy bones and tissues, but muscles in particular need oxygen to function properly and will benefit from regular outdoor exercise and from breathing deeply. Sometimes, a change to a healthy lifestyle can bring relief even to chronic skeletal and muscular problems, such as rheumatoid and osteo-arthritis. Essential oils may be used in addition to relax muscles, relieve pain, and cleanse and detoxify the system.

Cramp

Temporary muscular spasms during or after physical exertion are not uncommon, but a more long-term problem is the type of cramp that occurs in the evening or at night, affecting mainly the calf muscles and feet. Thought to be due to poor circulation or, possibly, calcium deficiency, this type of cramp can be effectively relieved by regular self-help aromatherapy treatment.

Useful Oils
Sweet marjoram, Roman chamomile, and mandarin can all help to relieve muscular spasms and prevent recurrence of cramp. Cypress is also reputed to be useful for its tonic properties.

Prevention
Bath Add *3 drops of sweet marjoram and 2 drops each of Roman chamomile and mandarin* to your bath every evening to relax you.
Application Mix the same blend of oils with *½fl oz (15ml/2½tsp) of carrier lotion or oil* and apply (page 21) nightly at first. Gradually reduce the application to every second night, then over the longer term, to twice weekly applications. If the cramp returns, increase the frequency of use.

Massage Ask a friend to give you a regular leg massage (pages 26 to 27), using the mix recommended under application.
Treatment
Application To relieve cramp, rub the area well, using the blend of oils recommended for preventative application, if you have them handy. Make a conscious effort also to relax your whole body.

Sprains

A sprain may occur when ligaments are torn or stretched by a sudden, jerky movement. The affected joint becomes swollen and painful. Sprains respond well to aromatherapy treatment. **Caution:** Be sure to seek medical attention if you think you have a broken or splintered bone.

Useful Oils
Sweet marjoram and rosemary are analgesic oils that will help to dull pain, while lavender is calming.

Treatment
Rest the affected joint as much as possible. If it is your ankle that is sprained, keep your foot up when resting and use a walking stick.

Foot or hand bath Add *4 drops of sweet marjoram and 2 drops of rosemary* to a bowl containing sufficient cold water to cover the joint. Mix well and soak the affected limb for no less than ten minutes.

Compress Use the same oils to make up a cold compress (page 21) and apply to the affected area immediately after the foot or hand bath, leaving for at least an hour.

Application Again use the same oils but mixed with *½fl oz (15ml/2½tsp) of carrier oil or lotion*. After removing the compress, gently stroke this mixture over the affected area.

Caution: Never massage a sprained joint. Apply a new compress every evening before bed and leave on overnight. Remove the following morning and apply the lotion or oil mixture. Continue with this treatment until the pain and swelling have disappeared.

Rheumatism and Arthritis

Rheumatism is a loose term which covers a variety of rheumatic and arthritic conditions, but is mainly used for those in which pain is experienced in the muscles. Arthritis is a term used to describe inflammation of the joints specifically; there are two main types. Rheumatoid arthritis is a chronic inflammation of the connective tissue around joints which causes pain, swelling, and stiffness, and is often accompanied by weight loss and tiredness. It seems to affect women more than men and, unlike osteo-arthritis, usually attacks pairs of joints. In severe cases, the joints can become crippled and deformed. Osteo-arthritis is a progressive wearing away of cartilage which results in severe pain and reduced mobility. The connective tissue thickens and fluid may fill the joint, causing swelling. Aromatherapy can help to relax muscles and relieve pain, but it cannot renew worn cartilage nor can it always help to relieve pain in the bone.

Useful Oils

In most cases, the same oils help both rheumatic and arthritic conditions. Where there is inflammation, Roman chamomile and/or lavender are helpful, while juniper berry, eucalyptus, cypress, lemon, and rosemary are all useful for reducing swelling. The warming properties of black pepper, sweet marjoram, and ginger help to relax muscles and relieve mild pain. For more severe pain, include Roman chamomile or cajuput for their analgesic properties.

Treatment

Diet A change in diet can often bring about a noticeable improvement. However, it is advisable to consult a nutritionist rather than to experiment with the wide range of diets available for rheumatism, since many of them are contradictory.

Bath Warm baths can help to relax muscles and relieve pain. Sprinkle *2 drops each of lavender and rosemary and 3 drops of eucalyptus* in the water. If pain is severe or persistent, add a further *2 drops of either cajuput or Roman chamomile*.

Compress Make up a warm compress (page 21) using the same oils with *3 drops of juniper berry* added. Place over affected areas and leave on overnight.

Application or Massage Use the *Calming and Anti-inflammatory Mix* below and apply regularly to affected areas. If you are able to lie flat, ask a friend to give you a full body massage (pages 24 to 30) using the same mix.

Caution: Apply only gentle pressure and avoid massage of painful or inflamed joints.

Calming and Anti-inflammatory Mix
5 drops each of juniper berry, eucalyptus, Roman chamomile, and lavender
2fl oz (60ml/10tsp) of carrier lotion or oil

Blend the essential oils and add to the carrier lotion or oil. Use the mix for application or for massage, as indicated.

77

Essential Oil of Roman Chamomile

Part of plant used: *Flowers*
Method of extraction: *Steam distillation*
Volatility: *Middle note (page 16)*
Principal constituent: *Esters (85%), azulene*

Properties, effects, and methods of use

Essential oil of Roman chamomile has multiple healing properties and a low toxicity that make it particularly suitable for use on children. It contains the powerful anti-inflammatory substance, azulene, which can relieve a wide variety of skin complaints. It has a light but sharp, apple-like aroma.

Emotional Calming and relaxing; relieves anxiety, stress, depression, hysteria, irritability, and neuralgia; helpful in overcoming headaches and insomnia; soothing for children's tantrums. Used in inhalations, vaporizers, baths, application, or massage.

Skin Soothing and antiseptic; good for sensitive and dry skins; helps to clear acne, eczema, diaper/nappy rash, burns, and minor wounds; reduces inflammation. Used in masks, compresses, application, or massage.

Digestive Antispasmodic and anti-inflammatory; soothes diarrhoea, constipation, indigestion, flatulence, and colic; restores appetite. Used in compresses, baths, application, or massage.

Muscular Calming and mild analgesic; soothes muscular aches and cramps due to physical exertion; relieves inflammation and pain in rheumatism and arthritis. Used in compresses, baths, application, or massage.

Gynaecological Soothing and antispasmodic; helps painful, heavy, or irregular menstruation; relieves pre-menstrual syndrome and menopausal symptoms. Used in compresses, baths, or application.

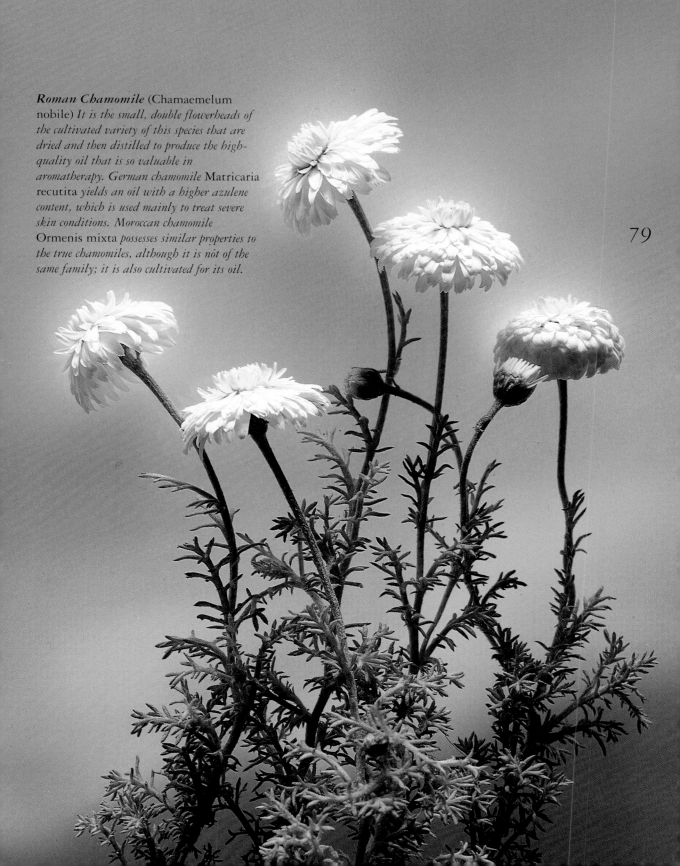

Roman Chamomile (Chamaemelum nobile) *It is the small, double flowerheads of the cultivated variety of this species that are dried and then distilled to produce the high-quality oil that is so valuable in aromatherapy.* German chamomile Matricaria recutita *yields an oil with a higher azulene content, which is used mainly to treat severe skin conditions.* Moroccan chamomile Ormenis mixta *possesses similar properties to the true chamomiles, although it is not of the same family; it is also cultivated for its oil.*

Gynaecological Problems

The menstrual cycle affects most women emotionally as well as physically every month, and with varying intensity. This is because menstruation is controlled by hormones released by the endocrine system, whose functioning is easily upset by stress (page 36). Aromatherapy is one of the most effective methods of treating menstrual and menopausal problems since many essential oils can help to regulate hormone production. Other relaxing and uplifting oils are useful for relieving the stress-related tension that often exacerbates symptoms. Taking regular exercise and eating a healthy, balanced diet (page 36) will further promote relaxation and increase the ability to cope with stress.

Pre-menstrual Syndrome (PMS)

Pre-menstrual syndrome may begin anytime between two to ten days before the onset of menstruation. Physical symptoms include excessive fluid retention in the breasts and abdomen, headaches, nausea, and facial spots. PMS may also involve extreme emotional reactions, such as intense irritability, depression and, very occasionally, violent behaviour. In many cases, symptoms appear to result from a stress-related hormonal imbalance, and respond well to preventative aromatherapy treatment.

Useful Oils

For emotional outbursts, lavender, true melissa, geranium, Roman chamomile, sandalwood, and rose otto are balancing to the emotions generally, while a combination of true melissa and clary sage will lift the spirits. If a headache (page 49) or fluid retention (page 72) is also a symptom, turn to the appropriate page and choose oils that are also recommended for stress on page 45.

Prevention

Begin any treatment for PMS well before you expect symptoms to start, even as early as three weeks before menstruation.

Diet Eat a healthy, balanced diet, drink only caffeine-free coffee, and avoid teas containing either caffeine or tannin (page 36). Dietary supplements of oil of evening primrose and vitamin B6 may be helpful, but you should keep to recommended dosages.

Treatment

Inhalation For rapid relief of headaches and emotional symptoms, sprinkle *2 drops each of true melissa, lavender, and Roman chamomile* on to a tissue and inhale deeply.

Massage Use the *Balancing and Relaxing Massage Mix* below and apply to the shoulders (page 31) or ask a friend to give you a whole body massage (pages 24 to 30).

Bath Add *3 drops of lavender and 2 drops of rose otto* to your bath to encourage relaxation. For details on treatments for fluid retention, see page 72; for pimples/spots, follow the guidelines given under acne on page 57.

Balancing and Relaxing Massage Mix
  4 drops each of clary sage and lavender
  2 drops of true melissa or rose otto
  1fl oz (30ml/5tsp) of carrier oil or lotion

Mix the essential oils with the carrier oil or lotion. Use for massage, as indicated.

Menstrual Pain

Menstrual pain affects a great many women immediately prior to, or during, the first day of bleeding, occasionally continuing into the second day. The pain, which is felt in the lower back and abdomen, is due to uterine cramping and may vary in severity from month to month, being exacerbated by a high level of stress (page 36) and too little time set aside for exercise and relaxation.
Caution: Where pain is persistent or very severe, consult a doctor, since this may indicate a more serious underlying problem.

Useful Oils

Clary sage, cypress, sweet marjoram, Roman chamomile, and rose otto are all good antispasmodics that help to reduce uterine cramping, while juniper berry is a useful cleanser and detoxifier. Sweet marjoram, rose otto, and Roman chamomile are also analgesics. Clary sage and true melissa are a good combination since the former is antispasmodic, the latter stimulating, and both are hormone regulators.

Prevention

Begin treatment at least ten days before menstruation is due.
Diet Supplements of calcium, magnesium, and vitamin B6 may prove helpful, but keep to recommended dosages.
Massage Add *2 drops each of rose otto, Roman chamomile, and cypress, and 4 drops of sweet marjoram to 1fl oz (30ml/5tsp) of carrier oil or lotion.* Apply nightly to the small of the back (page 32) and the lower abdomen. Or, ask a friend to massage the mixture into your back and abdomen (pages 25 and 30).

Treatment

Compress If you normally have to lie down due to the severity of the pain, a warm compress (page 21) containing *4 drops each of clary sage and sweet marjoram and 3 drops of Roman chamomile* may relieve cramping if applied to the lower back and abdomen.

Irregular Periods

Some women experience disconcerting irregularities in their menstrual cycle. Gaps between menstruation may vary from two to five weeks and, in extreme cases, as long as two months. Often, worry about the irregularity and doubts over the ability to conceive, may serve to aggravate symptoms. Regular aromatherapy treatment with soothing essential oils can do a lot to remedy this condition.
Caution: Seek medical advice if there is a total absence of menstruation.

Useful Oils

A combination of Roman chamomile, true melissa, and rose otto is particularly effective in regulating menstrual flow; the first two help to stimulate menstruation, while rose otto is a balancing oil. For a less costly alternative, combine rose otto with clary sage and lavender or juniper berry and rosemary. Peppermint is a useful decongestant.

Treatment

Application Add *2 drops each of rose otto, clary sage, and lavender and 3 drops of Roman chamomile to 1fl oz (30ml/5tsp) of carrier oil or lotion.* Apply to the abdomen and small of the back (page 32) on a daily basis to help reestablish your hormonal balance.
Bath Take regular baths, adding *a total of 8 drops* of a blend of the above recommended essential oils to the water.
Massage Ask a friend to give you a regular back, leg, and abdomen massage (pages 25, 26 to 27, and 30), using the *Massage Oil* below. Or, work the mixture into the small of the back (page 32) and the abdomen.

Regulating Massage Oil
 3 drops of rose otto and lavender
 2 drops each of true melissa and clary sage
 1 drop of Roman chamomile
 1fl oz (30ml/5tsp) of carrier oil

Mix the essential oils with the carrier oil. Use for massage, as indicated.

Essential Oil of Tea Tree

Part of plant used: *Leaves*
Method of extraction: *Steam distillation*
Volatility: *Top note (page 16)*
Principal constituents: *Terpenes, terpinolene, terpinen-4-ol, terpineol, cineole*

Properties, effects, and methods of use

Tea tree essential oil is an exceptionally powerful antiseptic, being 12 times as strong as carbolic acid, or phenol, the widely used chemical disinfectant. It has the advantage of being both hypo-allergenic and non-toxic, and it may also be effective against a range of bacterial, viral, and fungal conditions. The oil can be pale green to almost water clear, and its aroma is an effective insect repellant.

Respiratory Bactericidal and anti-viral; helps to fight colds and flu; alleviates sore throats, tonsillitis, and gum disease; eases bronchitis, chesty coughs, and congestion. Used in gargles, mouthwashes, compresses, inhalations, vaporizers, or application.

Skin Cleansing, cooling, and anti-fungal; effective against head lice; relieves boils and rashes; soothes sunburn; encourages open skin to heal while protecting it from infection; relieves athlete's foot and nailbed infections. Anti-parasitic; helps eliminate worms. Used in masks, compresses, foot or hand baths, or application.

Circulatory Tonic to veins; helps haemorrhoids and varicose veins.

Digestive Bactericidal, anti-viral, and anti-fungal; eases mouth ulcers, calms diarrhoea, and relieves gastroenteritis. Used in mouthwashes, compresses, application, or massage.

Gynaecological Anti-fungal; can help to clear vaginal thrush. Used in sitz baths, douches, baths, or application.

Caution Although tea tree is non-toxic at normal aromatherapy dosages, it contains cineole and is therefore regarded as toxic in Australia.

Tea Tree (Melaleuca alternifolia)
*When Captain Cook and his sailors first
visited the Australian continent, they are said
to have used the leaves of this tree to make a
refreshing hot drink. Whether or not they liked
the brew is uncertain, but the tree has kept the
name they gave it. Over the centuries, the
indigenous Aborigines have used tea tree
poultices to cleanse and heal wounds and
ulcers. Today tea tree is grown commercially
for its oil along the central and northern coasts
of New South Wales.*

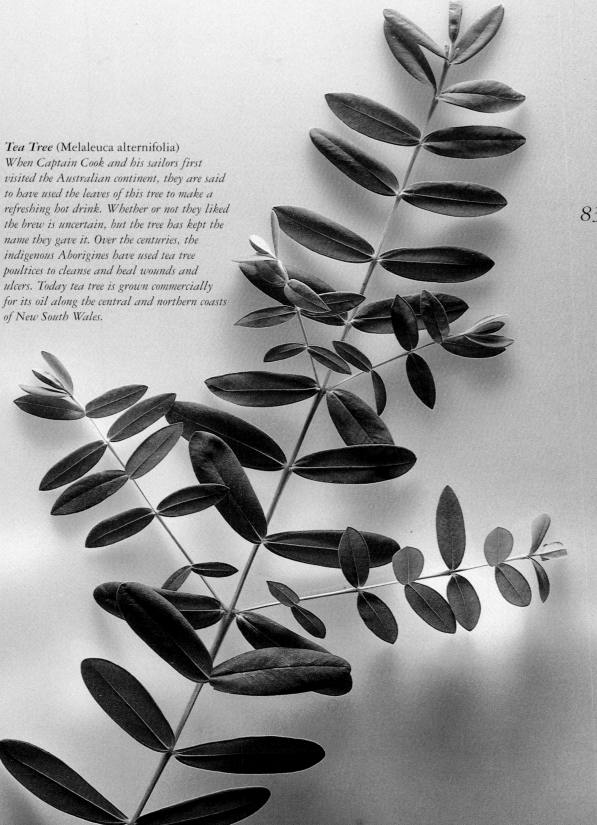

Vaginal Thrush

A yeast-like fungus *Candida albicans* lives naturally in our large intestine, its growth kept in check by beneficial bacteria. General poor health, a course of antibiotics, the contraceptive pill, pregnancy, and stress (page 36) may all upset the balance of friendly and harmful bacteria in your bowel, giving the *Candida* fungus the opportunity to multiply. Once out of control, the fungus can adversely affect the mucous lining of the vagina, occurring as a white, often smelly, discharge that is frequently accompanied by itching and inflammation. Vaginal thrush may respond well to treatment with antiseptic essential oils. **Caution:** If oral thrush develops, consult your doctor, since this may indicate a more serious immunocomprised condition.

Useful Oils

Tea tree, myrrh, and lavender have anti-fungal properties that may relieve thrush. Lavender also improves the aroma of a mix.

Treatment

Diet Eating plenty of live natural yoghurt will help to restore the balance of bacteria in your bowel; fresh, raw garlic and onion are also recommended. Avoid alcohol, coffee, refined carbohydrates, and yeasty or sugary foods and drinks. Any of these can contribute to the imbalance in intestinal flora and encourage the harmful fungi to multiply.

Bath Sprinkle *6 drops of tea tree and 2 drops of myrrh* into a warm bath. Kneel down in the bath and swish the water several times on to the vaginal area before sitting down. Remain sitting for at least ten minutes.

Tampon application Tea tree is a mild oil, despite its powerful aroma, and may be used undiluted for vaginal insertion following an allergy test (page 19). **Caution:** No other oil may be used in this way. Apply *2 drops of neat tea tree oil* to the top of a damp tampon and insert into your vagina. Leave in place for three to four hours.

Application Use the *Anti-fungal Mix* below to soothe the outer areas of the vagina.

Anti-fungal Mix
  2 drops of myrrh
  4 drops of lavender
  ¹/₂fl oz (15ml2¹/₂tsp) of carrier lotion or oil

Mix the essential oils with carrier lotion or oil and use for application, as indicated.

Menopausal Problems

The menopause is a normal and natural part of the ageing process, covering the period during which menstruation slows down and eventually ceases to exist. It can occur any-time from the early forties to middle fifties, but on average begins around 50 years of age. It is due to hormonal changes, in particular a gradual reduction in the production of oestrogen and progesteron. Some women are lucky and notice only a reduction in flow or a gradual lengthening of the periods between menstruation. Others are less fortunate and experience some of the more unpleasant symptoms associated with this condition, of which the two most common are hot flashes/flushes and depression. Either of these two symptoms may be triggered or aggravated by stress (page 36).

Useful Oils

Essential oils that regulate hormone production include lemon, pine, bitter orange, sandalwood, lavender, cypress, clary sage, geranium, and the three commonly favoured for "women's problems" – rose otto, Roman chamomile, and true melissa. For relief of hot flashes/flushes, one of these three oils may be combined with clary sage or sandalwood, with peppermint added for its cooling qualities. If you are depressed (page 45), turn to the appropriate page and choose an oil such as clary sage or true melissa that contains both uplifting and hormone-regulating properties.

Treatment

Hormone replacement therapy may be recommended, particularly where a future risk of bone deterioration (osteoporosis) is indicated, but be wary of this treatment since it can have unwanted side effects.

Lifestyle Set aside time for exercise and relaxation, and make a conscious effort to be positive in your approach to life. If you can, keep away from hot or stressful environments since either may bring on hot flashes/flushes.

Diet Avoid spicy foods and alcohol. Drink peppermint tea regularly for its cooling qualities, and include calcium-rich dairy foods (or sesame-seed products if you are vegetarian) to help prevent bone deterioration.

Inhalation To help relieve a hot flash/flush, sprinkle *a few drops of peppermint* on to a tissue and inhale deeply. You can also carry a bottle of peppermint oil around with you for use, as indicated, whenever you feel the symptoms coming on.

Gargle To alleviate a hot flash/flush, add *2 drops of peppermint or lemon to ½ a glass of water* and gargle (page 21) with the mixture.

Bath To prevent recurrence of symptoms, sprinkle *3 drops of clary sage and 2 drops each of rose otto and peppermint* into a daily bath.

Massage Ask a friend to give you a whole body massage (pages 24 to 30) once or twice a week on a regular basis, using the *Hormone-regulating Massage Oil* below. Alternatively, use the same blend of oils diluted in *1fl oz (30ml/5tsp) of carrier lotion* and massage daily into your shoulders (page 31) and the small of your back. For depression, turn to page 45 for advice on appropriate treatments to use.

Hormone-regulating Massage Oil
    2 drops each of rose otto and sandalwood
    3 drops each of bitter orange and cypress
    1fl oz (30ml/5tsp) of carrier oil

Mix the essential oils with the carrier oil. Use for massage, as indicated.

Cystitis

Cystitis is an inflammation of the bladder lining. It can result from infection or from a build up of irritant toxic substances in the urine which are ingested in food. Sexual intercourse can also cause irritation. Cystitis is not a gynaecological problem but it is included here since women are more often affected than men. Symptoms may include an urge to urinate when there is no need and a painful burning sensation prior to, during, and, sometimes, after passing urine. Cystitis can be mild or severe and may recur, but it can be speedily curtailed if treated at the onset.

Caution: If cystitis is accompanied by fever or back pain, consult a doctor, since this can indicate a kidney infection.

Useful Oils

Juniper berry, cajuput, eucalyptus, pine, and sandalwood are helpful antiseptic oils. Juniper berry is also a useful detoxifier, while sandalwood can ease irritation.

Treatment

Lifestyle Wash the external area around your bladder exit with water rather than soap, and after urinating, wipe from front to rear.

Diet Drink plenty of fluids and eat a healthy diet (page 36), avoiding refined or processed foods. Include plenty of garlic and onion.

Bath Sprinkle *2 drops each of juniper berry, eucalyptus, and sandalwood* into a warm bath. Kneel down in the bath and swish the water on to the affected area. Repeat several times, then sit in the water for ten minutes.

Application Use the *Astringent, Soothing Mix* below and apply to the external area of the bladder. Repeat two or three times a day.

Astringent, Soothing Mix
    2 drops each of juniper berry and eucalyptus
    2 drops of sandalwood
    ½fl oz (15ml/2½tsp) of carrier oil or lotion

Mix the essential oils with the carrier oil or lotion. Use for application, as indicated.

Essential Oil of Sandalwood

Part of plant used: *Wood*
Method of extraction: *Steam distillation*
Volatility: *Base note (page 16)*
Principal constituents: *Santalol (over 90%)*

Properties, effects, and methods of use

Sandalwood essential oil is profoundly calming and soothing in effect. It is also an excellent antiseptic for both pulmonary and urinary systems. The oil has a rich woody smell, which makes it pleasant for therapeutic use.

Emotional Sedative and relaxing; beneficial for relieving anxiety, tension, and lifting depression; helpful in freeing the mind from the past; invaluable as a remedy for insomnia. Used in inhalations, vaporizers, baths, application, or massage.

Respiratory Soothing and antiseptic; relieves irritation and soreness in chesty coughs, sore throats, and laryngitis; soothes bronchitis and asthma. Used in gargles, inhalations, vaporizers, application, or massage.

Skin Balancing and decongestant; softens dry, mature, or wrinkled skin; helps dry dandruff and eczema; may help to reduce irritation from sunburn, nettle rash, hives, diaper/nappy rash, and allergic conditions. Used in compresses, application, or massage.

Digestive Calming and astringent; subdues vomiting, colic, and hiccups; helpful for diarrhoea; soothes heartburn and nausea, especially morning sickness. Used in compresses, application, or massage.

Circulatory Soothing; relieves itchiness and congestion in haemorrhoids and varicose veins. Used in compresses or application.

Gynaecological Calming and balancing; may be helpful for pre-menstrual and menopausal symptoms; also for impotence. Used in baths or application.

Sandalwood oil is anti-infections and soothes cystitits when used in baths or application.

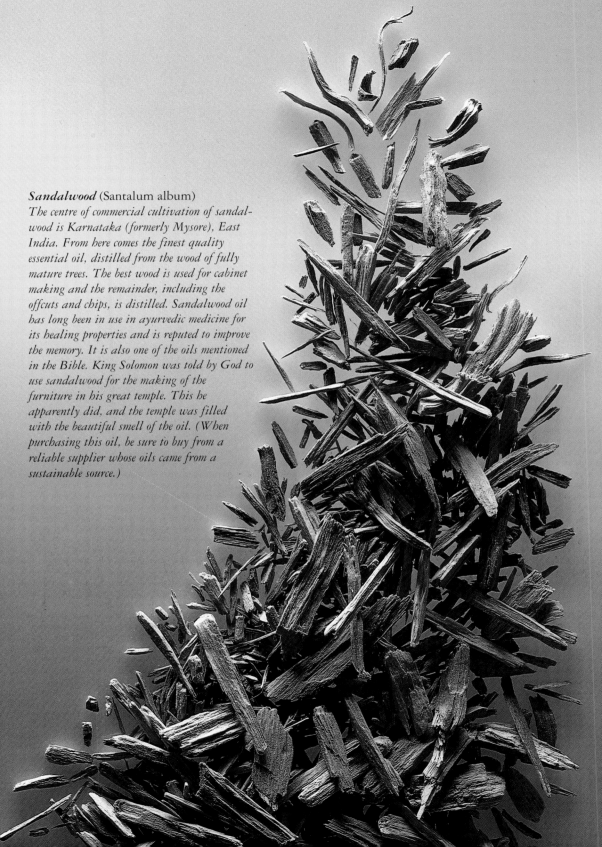

Sandalwood (Santalum album)

The centre of commercial cultivation of sandal-wood is Karnataka (formerly Mysore), East India. From here comes the finest quality essential oil, distilled from the wood of fully mature trees. The best wood is used for cabinet making and the remainder, including the offcuts and chips, is distilled. Sandalwood oil has long been in use in ayurvedic medicine for its healing properties and is reputed to improve the memory. It is also one of the oils mentioned in the Bible. King Solomon was told by God to use sandalwood for the making of the furniture in his great temple. This he apparently did, and the temple was filled with the beautiful smell of the oil. (When purchasing this oil, be sure to buy from a reliable supplier whose oils came from a sustainable source.)

Children's Problems

During the first few months of your child's life, stomach upsets and minor skin disorders, such as diaper/nappy rash, are common health problems that may be encountered. Cuts and bruises are likely as your child begins to walk and explore and, once at school, he or she may be exposed to a range of infectious diseases. Aromatherapy can be a highly effective preventative measure, both in its role as an immune-system booster and because of the gentle cleansing qualities of many of the oils. To be effective, however, it needs to be combined with a healthy lifestyle and diet (page 36). Children also need to feel loved in order to thrive and here regular aromatherapy massage can be extremely beneficial.

Points to Observe

○ For children of more than three years old, use half the number of drops recommended for adults.

○ For children of less than three years of age, use quarter the number of drops recommended for adults. When bathing babies of under 18 months, add only one drop of essential oil to the water, swishing well to disperse.

○ Keep all essential oils out of the reach of children.

○ Keep all essential oils, whether neat or diluted, away from your child's eyes.

○ Only allow your child to apply a ready mixed lotion or oil when properly supervised.

○ Inhalations should be used on children only for a short period. Never allow your child near a bowl of hot water in which essential oils are diluted, unless properly supervised.

○ Use only the 12 oils featured in this chapter. **Caution:** Keep to the dilutions specified and follow any cautionary advice closely.

○ Before treating your child, read the Points to Observe on page 43, chapter 2 How to Use Home Treatments (in particular the Points to Observe on page 19), and the cautions on the use of essential oils on page v.

Infantile Colic

The term "infantile colic" is used to describe the bouts of stomach pain that commonly affect babies during their first few months. When a bout occurs, your baby may cry continuously, even when picked up. The pain may come in waves over several hours and may recur at regular times every day. In addition to indigestion, a variety of factors are thought to give rise to colic and if attacks are recurrent or prolonged, consult a doctor.

Useful Oils

Roman chamomile and juniper berry will help release gas, while sweet marjoram and sandalwood will relax spasms and stimulate the digestion.

Prevention

Try to ensure that your baby does not drink too quickly or take in air with the milk, and burp/wind him or her after every feed.

Treatment

Massage Mix *2 drops each of sweet marjoram and Roman chamomile* with *2fl oz (60ml/10tsp) of carrier lotion or oil.* When colic occurs after feeding, use this mixture sparingly to massage your baby's tummy gently for a few minutes. Work in a clockwise direction.

Head Lice

The head louse is a small, flat, wingless insect that infests the scalp and sometimes the eyebrows and eyelashes, laying its eggs along the base of the hair shafts. The head louse feeds by sucking blood from the scalp and its bite may itch severely and sometimes become infected. Infestation is common in children and easily transmitted through direct head contact or use of the same comb, towel, or headgear. If there is an outbreak at your child's school, check for infestation by examining the hair shafts near the scalp for eggs. You can also run a fine-toothed comb through your child's hair every evening over the bath to check for the presence of adult lice.

Useful Oils

Eucalyptus, geranium, and lavender are antiseptics that may be effective in relieving this condition.

Treatment

Application Add *2 drops of eucalyptus and 1 drop each of lavender and geranium to 1 tsp of carrier lotion.* Massage the mix into the scalp and leave for half an hour. Run a fine-toothed comb through the hair before shampooing, and then wash and rinse well. Finally, apply the *Antiseptic Rinse* below, carefully pouring the mixture over the whole head so that it covers every hair. Leave to dry naturally. Repeat daily until both lice and eggs have disappeared. As a preventative measure against further infestation, use the same mixture as a final rinse every time you wash your child's hair. **Caution:** Be careful to keep any essential oil mix out of your child's eyes.

Antiseptic Rinse
> *2 drops each of eucalyptus, lavender, rosemary, and geranium*
> *½fl oz (15ml/2½tsp) of vinegar*
> *8fl oz (240ml) of water*

Blend the oils, vinegar, and water for application, as indicated, stirring well before use.

Diaper/Nappy Rash

Diaper/nappy rash affects most babies at one time or another, occurring as a red rash around the areas closest to where urine is excreted. It may be caused by wet or soiled diapers/nappies, and in some cases a fungal infection may superimpose itself on the rash, causing flesh to become raw and painful.

Useful Oils

Tea tree is highly antiseptic and may be used regularly to disinfect diapers/nappies. For your baby's skin, oils such as sandalwood, lavender, and Roman chamomile, diluted in calendula carrier oil, are soothing. Lavender, in particular, has the ability to heal broken skin by stimulating cell renewal.

Prevention

Apply the *Lotion* from the recipe to your baby's bottom at each diaper/nappy change.

Treatment

Lifestyle Change diapers/nappies frequently, each time leaving your baby's bottom exposed to the fresh air for a few minutes. Instead of using a proprietary brand of disinfectant, soak washable diapers/nappies in a bucket of water containing *8 drops of tea tree.* When washing them, use only a small amount of powder to avoid leaving a potentially irritant residue. Add *2 drops of lavender* oil to a final hand rinse, or *6 drops* to the softening agent in the rinse programme of your washing machine.

Application Use the soothing recipe below and apply sparingly and gently to your baby's bottom at each diaper/nappy change.

Soothing Baby Oil or Lotion
> *4 drops of lavender*
> *2 drops of Roman chamomile*
> *1 drop of sandalwood*
> *2fl oz (60ml/10tsp) of calendula carrier oil or lotion*

Mix the essential oils with the carrier oil or lotion and use for application, as indicated.

Essential Oil of Lavender

Part of plant used: *Flowering tops*
Method of extraction: *Steam distillation*
Volatility: *Middle note (page 16)*
Principal constituents: *Linalyl and geranyl esters, geraniol, linalol*

Properties, effects, and methods of use

Lavender essential oil has a balancing and normalizing effect, bringing health and harmony to body and mind. It is non-toxic, and has a full, flowery aroma.

Emotional Uplifting and soothing; alleviates stress, anxiety, depression, and general debility; helpful for insomnia, headaches, and migraine. Used in inhalations, vaporizers, compresses, baths, application, or massage.

Respiratory Antiseptic and anti-inflammatory; eases colds, flu, sinusitis, and throat infections. Used in inhalations, vaporizers, baths, or application.

Skin Balancing, antiseptic, anti-inflammatory, and regenerative; soothes acne, eczema, dandruff, hair loss, diaper/nappy nash, sunburn, insect bites, and boils; relieves athlete's foot; effective for burns and stretchmarks since it promotes cell growth and helps to minimize scarring. Used in masks, compresses, baths, or application.

Digestive Cleansing and calming; helps bad breath, mouth ulcers, indigestion, flatulence, nausea, and gastroenteritis. Used in compresses, gargles, application, or massage.

Circulatory Hypotensive; lowers blood pressure; reduces palpitations; may alleviate fluid retention. Used in baths, application, or massage.

Muscular Analgesic and anti-inflammatory; helpful for muscular sprains, aches, pains, and rheumatism. Used in compresses, baths, application, or massage.

Gynaecological Calming and balancing; helps to establish menstrual regularity; good for pre-menstrual and menopausal symptoms; alleviates thrush. Used in compresses, inhalations, vaporizers, baths, or application.

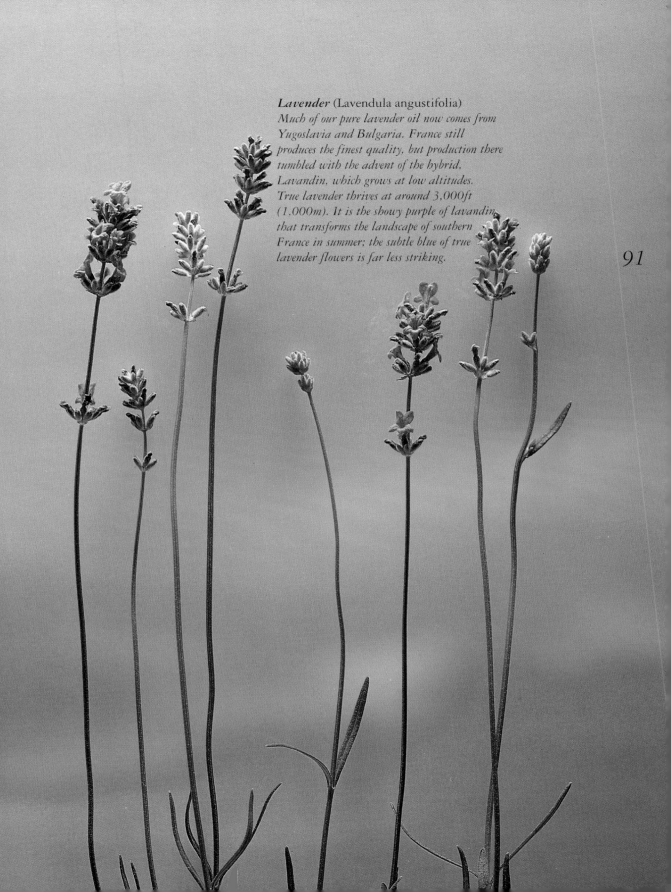

Lavender (Lavendula angustifolia)
Much of our pure lavender oil now comes from
Yugoslavia and Bulgaria. France still
produces the finest quality, but production there
tumbled with the advent of the hybrid,
Lavandin, which grows at low altitudes.
True lavender thrives at around 3,000ft
(1,000m). It is the showy purple of lavandin
that transforms the landscape of southern
France in summer; the subtle blue of true
lavender flowers is far less striking.

First Aid

Essential oils are natural cleansers and gentle healers and it is certainly worth reorganizing your first-aid kit to accommodate them. A basic kit should include the following items: a large and a small bandage, a pair of scissors, tweezers, plasters, adhesive tape, cotton balls/cotton wool, gauze, and a piece of cotton cloth for a compress. To these, add a small measuring cup or eggcup for mixing oils, a 2fl oz (60ml) bottle of carrier oil or lotion, and the following selection of essential oils: geranium, lavender, Roman chamomile, sweet marjoram, and tea tree.

Points to Observe
○ Never attempt self-diagnosis. If you are unsure of the cause, nature, or severity of an injury or ailment, you should seek medical advice immediately.
○ Make up only small quantities of ready-prepared mixes, and label them clearly.
○ Secure your first-aid box with a firm catch, but no lock, and store it well out of reach of children.

Insect Bites and Stingers/Stings
If a wasp or bee stinger/sting is left in the skin, remove it carefully with tweezers.
Treatment
Application Apply *1 drop each of lavender and tea tree* to the stinger/sting or bite. Repeat at hourly intervals until irritation ceases. For subsequent applications, use *4 drops of lavender and tea tree* diluted in *1 tsp of carrier oil or lotion.* Apply twice daily until symptoms have cleared. **Caution:** Some people may be extremely sensitive to insect bites and stingers/stings and suffer an acute reaction, in which case seek medical attention immediately. If you are stung in the mouth, nose, or throat or if the area is painful again after a few days, consult a doctor.

Minor Burns
Hold a minor burn under running cold water for 10 minutes, unless the skin is broken.
Treatment
Application Apply *lavender oil* immediately to the affected area. If you wish to use a piece of gauze to cover it, secure it only at the edges, with adhesive tape. Repeat the application every two hours for 24 hours, without removing the gauze. If the burn has not healed, dilute *6 drops of lavender and 2 drops of geranium* in *1 tsp of carrier oil.* Apply the mix to the affected area. Repeat four times a day until it has healed. **Caution:** Seek medical attention if the burn is severe.

Minor Bruises
Keep the mix below ready prepared for use.
Treatment
Application Mix *15 drops of sweet marjoram and 8 drops each of geranium and Roman chamomile* with *1fl oz (30ml/5tsp) of calendula oil or lotion.* Apply immediately. Repeat every hour until no longer painful to the touch. If a bruise does form, apply the same mix every two hours until it diminishes. **Caution:** If there is swelling, seek medical advice.

Glossary of Therapeutic Terms

Explanations of principal therapeutic properties are given below, together with the oils to which they are commonly attributed. For details on healing effects that are believed to be common to all essential oils, see page 16.

analgesic (pain-relieving) Cajeput, Ginger, Lavender, Roman Chamomile, Rosemary, Rose Otto, Sweet Marjoram, True Melissa

anti-fungal (arresting growth of fungi or mould) Geranium, Lavender, Lemon, Myrrh, Tagetes, Tea Tree

anti-inflammatory (reducing inflammation) Clary Sage, Eucalyptus, Lavender, Peppermint, Petitgrain, Roman Chamomile, Rose Otto, Sandalwood

antispasmodic (preventing or relieving muscular cramps or convulsions) Clary Sage, Cypress, Mandarin, Peppermint, Roman Chamomile, Rosemary, Rose Otto, Sandalwood, Sweet Marjoram

anti-viral (destroying viral activity) Black Pepper, Geranium, Lemon, Tea Tree

astringent (contracting body tissues and reducing secretions) Cypress, Geranium, Juniper Berry, Lemon, Peppermint, Rosemary, Sandalwood

balancing (restoring, or maintaining, a state of equilibrium) most essential oils but particularly Atlas Cedarwood, Clary Sage, Geranium, Juniper Berry, Lavender, Lemon, Roman Chamomile, Rosemary, Rose Otto, Sandalwood, True Melissa, Ylang Ylang

carminative (expelling of gas/wind from stomach) Caraway, Juniper Berry, Ginger, Mandarin, Peppermint, Rosemary

cleansing (clearing impurities) Atlas Cedarwood, Cajeput, Geranium, Juniper Berry, Lavender, Lemon, Peppermint, Pine, Rosemary, Tea Tree

decongestant (reducing congestion) Atlas Cedarwood, Eucalyptus, Lavender, Patchouli, Peppermint, Pine, Rosemary

digestive (stimulating the digestive process) Black Pepper, Bitter Orange, Caraway, Ginger, Juniper Berry, Lavender, Lemon, Mandarin, Sweet Marjoram, Peppermint, Roman Chamomile, Rosemary

diuretic (increasing flow of urine) Juniper Berry, Lavender, Rosemary

emmenagogic (inducing menstruation) Clary Sage, Lavender, Roman Chamomile, Rosemary, Sweet Marjoram, True Melissa

hormone regulator (regulating hormone production) Bitter Orange, Clary Sage, Cypress, Lavender, Lemon, Pine, Roman Chamomile, Rose Otto, Sandalwood, True Melissa

regenerative (stimulating healthy growth and renewal of cells) most essential oils but particularly Frankincense, Lavender, Myrrh

relaxing Clary Sage, Geranium, Juniper Berry, Lavender, Lemon, Mandarin, Neroli, Petitgrain, Roman Chamomile, Rose Otto, Sandalwood, Sweet Marjoram, True Melissa, Ylang Ylang

stimulating (increasing activity) Black Pepper, Bitter Orange, Geranium, Juniper Berry, Lemon, Peppermint, Roman Chamomile, Rosemary, True Melissa, Ylang Ylang

soothing (relieving irritation) Clary Sage, Cypress, Geranium, Lavender, Peppermint, Roman Chamomile, Sandalwood, Sweet Marjoram

uplifting Clary Sage, Eucalyptus, Geranium, Juniper Berry, Lavender, Petitgrain, Roman Chamomile, Rosemary, Rose Otto, Sandalwood, True Melissa, Ylang Ylang

Further Reading

Chaitow, L. *The Body/Mind Purification Program* (Simon & Schuster, 1990)

Davis, P. *Aromatherapy: an A-Z* (C W Daniel, UK, 1988)

Monro, Dr R., Nagarathna, Dr., and Nagendra, Dr. *Yoga for Common Ailments* (Simon & Schuster, 1990)

Price, Shirley *Practical Aromatherapy* (revised edition, Thorsons, UK, 1987)

Stanway, P. *Foods for Common Ailments* (Simon & Schuster, 1989)

Thomas, S. *Massage for Common Ailments* (Simon & Schuster, 1989)

Tisserand, R. *The Art of Aromatherapy* (Inner Traditions, 1978) and *Aromatherapy for Everyone* (revised edition, Penguin, UK, 1990)

Useful Addresses

Suppliers and mail-order distributors of quality, pure essential oils, carrier oils and lotions, and aromatherapy skin-care products. Those addresses marked with an asterik also supply vaporizers.

Body Essentials, 108 Central Avenue, Westfield, NJ 07090. Tel: 201 322 5099

*Bonne Sante Health Products, 642 62nd Street, Brooklyn, NY 11220, USA. Tel: 718 492 3887

Margot Latimer, PO Box 65, Pineville, PA 18946, USA. Tel: 215 598 3802

Julia Meadows, 323 E. Matilija 112, Ojai, CA 93023, USA. Tel: 805 640 1300.

Just Good Scents Co Ltd., 20b Collingwood Court, Edmonton, Alberta T5T OH5, Canada. Tel: 416 897 7120

LNJ Trading, 844 North Star Mall, San Antonio TX 78216, USA. Tel: 512 341 1709

Swedish Health Care Center, 178 Milcreek Road, Livingston, MT 59047. Tel: 406 333 4216

The S.E.E.D. Institute, 3170 Kirwin Avenue, No 605 Mississauga, Ontario L5A 3R1, Canada. Tel: 416 897 7120

For information about essential oils, training courses, and qualified practitioners in your area, contact the following:

Margot Latimer, PO Box 65, Pineville, PA 18946, USA. Tel: 215 598 3802

Julia Meadows, 323 E. Matilija 112, Ojai, CA 93023, USA. Tel: 805 640 1300

The International Society of Professional Aromatherapists (ISPA), 41 Leicester Road, Hinckley, Leics LE10 1LW, England. Tel: 0455 637987

Buying and Storing Essential Oils and Carriers

○ Only buy neat essential oils if they are stocked in $^1/_4$ or $^1/_2$ fl oz (7 or 15ml) brown-glass bottles and clearly labelled "pure essential oil".

○ At home, store your essential oils and ready-prepared mixes in a cool, dark place and make sure the tops of the bottles are firmly secured. Heat, light, and air all detract from the therapeutic powers of an essential oil.

○ When correctly stored, distilled essential oils will keep for several years, but expressed oils are best used within six months.

○ Cold-pressed vegetable-oil carriers keep for up to six months if stored in the fridge. Remove several hours before needed.

○ Use oil-based mixes within nine months; lotion-based mixes will last for longer.

Index

94

95

Author's acknowledgments
I would like to thank my husband Len for his invaluable research assistance, and for his patience and understanding during the writing of this book – in the car, on aeroplanes, and even during meals! My thanks go to all my staff, who have had to manage without me, or suffer me under stress. They have been wonderful. Thanks are also due to my son Matthew and daughter Penny, both of whom have given me their help when needed. To Gian, who has had to keep me within page limits, I give my very warm thanks for her patience. My gratitude also to Helen for her inspired approach to photography and artistic layout. The medical readers, in particular, deserve thanks for their helpful suggestions.

Publisher's acknowledgments
The publishers would like to thank the following: Philip Dowell, Fausto Dorelli, Ann Chasseaud, Jeremy Gunn-Taylor; Dr Richard James, Dr George Bennett, and Dr Richard Donze for checking the manuscript; Libby Hoseason for guidance and support; Fiona Trent for proofreading; Lesley Gilbert for copy preparation; Michele Staple for compiling the index; Lynette Beckford and Lesley Causon for posing for photography; and Mildred Durne of Westhall Herbs, Kathleen Bagan, Kay Barr, Glasgow Botanic Gardens, and Wisley Gardens for plants. Special thanks are also due to Joss Pearson, Bridget Morley, Jonathan Hilton, Sara Mathews, Phil Gamble, Susan Walby, Alison Jones, Imogen Bright, Odile Lollis-Sydney, and Samantha Nunn.